Penguin Books
SHOW ME YOURS!
Understanding Children's Sexuality

Ronald Goldman is Foundation Professor of Education at La Trobe University in Australia and former Principal of Didsbury College of Education in England. His publications include *Religious Thinking from Childhood to Adolescence* (1964), *Readiness for Religion* (1965), *Breakthrough* (1968) and *Angry Adolescence* (1969). In 1982, he co-authored *Children's Sexual Thinking* with Juliette Goldman.

Juliette Goldman has several years experience as an infant and primary school teacher. She is a graduate in Sociology from the Australian National University and has a doctorate from La Trobe University. In 1982 she published *Children's Sexual Thinking* in conjunction with her husband and has contributed to various educational journals.

SHOW ME YOURS!

Understanding Children's Sexuality

RONALD AND JULIETTE GOLDMAN

PENGUIN BOOKS

Penguin Books Australia Ltd,
487 Maroondah Highway, P.O. Box 257
Ringwood, Victoria 3134, Australia
Penguin Books Ltd,
Harmondsworth, Middlesex, England
Viking-Penguin
40 West 23rd Street, New York, N.Y. 10010, U.S.A.
Penguin Books Canada Limited,
2801 John Street, Markham, Ontario, Canada L3R 1B4
Penguin Books (N.Z.) Ltd,
182-190 Wairau Road, Auckland 10, New Zealand

First published by Penguin Books Australia, 1988

Typeset in Garamond in 10 pt by Midland Typesetters, Maryborough, Vic.
Made and printed in Australia by Australian Print Group

CIP

Goldman, Ronald, 1922-   .
Show me yours! Understanding children's
sexuality.

Includes index.
ISBN 0 14 010714 2.

1. Children and sex. I. Goldman, Juliette.
II. Title.

155.4'18

Dedicated to Mary Calderone and David Finkelhor,
two pioneers who made this book possible

CONTENTS

PREFACE   xi

INTRODUCTION: CHILDREN ARE SEXUAL   xvii

PART ONE
WHAT CHILDREN THINK ABOUT SEX

1   HOW SEX DIFFERENCES ARE PERCEIVED   5

2   HOW ARE BABIES MADE?   21

3   WHAT HAPPENS IN PREGNANCY
AND CHILDBIRTH?   38

4   SEXUAL INTERCOURSE AND SEX
DETERMINATION   58

5   HOW NOT TO HAVE BABIES   71

6   WEARING CLOTHES AND BEING NAKED   89

7   WHAT THE YOUNG WANT TO KNOW ABOUT SEX   102

PART TWO
CHILDREN'S SEXUAL EXPERIENCES

8   PARENTS AND MARRIAGE   123

9   SEXUAL EMBARRASSMENTS IN THE FAMILY   137

10   CHILDREN WITH OTHER CHILDREN:
CURIOSITY AND EXPLORATION   148

11   CHILDREN WITH ADULTS:
CHILD SEXUAL ABUSE   164

12   CHILDREN WITH RELATIVES: INCEST   180

13   FIRST SEXUAL EXPERIENCES   195

PART THREE
WHAT DOES IT ALL MEAN?

14 HELPING ADULTS TO HELP CHILDREN 215

15 SOME DIFFICULT AND UNRESOLVED ISSUES 235

NOTES AND REFERENCES 254

INDEX 263

ACKNOWLEDGMENTS

We are greatly indebted to the principals and staff of schools in Australia, Britain, Canada, Sweden and the United States, and of the many Australian tertiary institutions from which we drew the students involved in our studies. In particular we are grateful to the university Schools of Education in several countries which we used as a base from which to contact schools. We are especially grateful to Dr Gunilla Westin-Lindgren who graciously organised the Swedish sample of children in our first study. Support also came from Dr David Finkelhor, who granted permission for us to use his interview schedule pioneered at the University of New Hampshire, USA, which formed the basis of our second study.

Neither study would have been possible without the financial assistance of the Australian Research Grants Scheme, the Swedish National Board of Education, the La Trobe University School of Education Research Committee and La Trobe's Centre for the Study of Community, Education and Social Change.

Because of the international aspect of the studies we undertook, an enormous amount of work was involved in correspondence, filing, documentation and manuscript typing, for which we express our immeasurable gratitude to Pauline Church, Mary Sepe and Maria Palmieri. And for advice and programming on the very demanding statistical analysis we are indebted to Mrs Di Worrell, Dr Glenn Rowley and Dr Daryl Caulley.

Last, but certainly not least, we express our thanks to more than two thousand school children and tertiary students who provided their ideas and views on sexuality. By their participation in our studies they have, we believe, provided newer insights and more realistic guidelines for helping future students to a happier and healthier sexual growth.

PREFACE

'Getting married means you can have more sex relations.' (What does that mean?) 'Oh, you can have more aunts and uncles' (English boy, 9 years).
'The hospital people get the hair and bones and things, they get them from girl bodies if they want to make a girl' (Australian boy, 7 years).
'Pregnancy? That's a night club in New York' (American girl, 9 years).

It is interesting, as well as amusing, to see how children use and misuse sexual words, to find out what they know about conception, childbirth and marriage, and to know what their earliest sexual experiences are.

Most children up to the age of 11, for example, because they have never had a satisfactory explanation about how a baby is born, believe that all babies are born by Caesarean section. In reality the figure for children born by this method in Australia is between 12% and 16%. But because they have heard so much talk about it and can think of no aperture wide enough in the mother's body by which a baby may be born, they end up thinking that cutting open the mother is necessary for all babies.

Younger children have even developed a Caesarean theory of conception. Because sexual intercourse is a secret from which most adults protect them, many children explain babies inside the mother in terms of a miniature baby being implanted in her at the clinic or the hospital. How is this done? By the baby being made out of the recycled hair, skin, bones and teeth of the people who die there. Then mother is cut open and after the tiny baby has been inserted, she is stitched up (sometimes zipped up) and several minutes, hours, months or years later opened up again for the fully grown baby to emerge. Mother is seen by many as some kind of extra fast microwave oven. This may seem fantastic and unusual, but children provide plenty of evidence that in the absence of accurate explanations they will invent their own. Some of the myths they create are perfectly logical, given the incomplete pieces of the sexual jigsaw they set out to put together. Like primitive peoples, they develop these myths to interpret what they do not understand. Much ingenuity, complexity and creativity are expressed in these sexual myths, opening up a whole new fascinating aspect of how children think.

But more important questions about children's sexuality need to be asked. How do children really respond to a new baby in the family? Do children understand anything about their parents' sexuality? How are they trained to be modest in their dress and how soon do they develop inhibitions about being seen naked? How prevalent is early masturbation, and what proportion of children indulge in sex games with their peers? More important, what is the prevalence of child sexual abuse and is it true that children are in greater sexual danger from adults they know, including members of their own family, than from strangers?

THE BASIS FOR THIS BOOK

What children think about and experience sexually is not a matter for guesswork. The rhymes and sayings of children have been documented in several books showing that children may know more than adults care to admit, although the sexual nature of what they are singing is often heavily disguised.

Old King Cole had a forty foot pole
And he showed it to the lady next door;
She thought it was a snake and hit it with a rake
And now it's only two foot four. [1]

Children's folklore does give us a useful glimpse of how children think, or would wish to think, about sex. But we need more than glimpses. There is now a more substantial and systematic body of knowledge about childhood sexuality which can help all who have to deal with children. Parents, teachers, psychologists, psychiatrists, pediatricians, the medical and other helping professions, need a straightforward account of what is known in this area. Talk or behaviour which might otherwise cause undue anxiety may not be a problem if normal sexual development can be seen objectively. What we should do for our children will become clearer if we understand the ways in which children think, behave and experience sexually.

Curiously, until recent times we knew more about the sexual pathologies of childhood than about normality. Much has been written about the Oedipal complex, about child pornography and intra-familial sexual abuse or incest, but relatively little about the more typical experiences of most children.

This book is an attempt to provide perspectives on the normal sexual development of children by presenting two kinds of evidence. The first kind is the now accepted views of the experts, the body of knowledge accumulated over the last few decades or more, based upon a great deal of research and clinical evidence. This is covered mainly in this book's Introduction, 'Children are Sexual'.

Most of the book, however, describes the researches of the authors over the past few years. Our first study involved interviews with almost 1000 children aged 5 to 15 in five countries – Australia, the USA, Canada, England and Sweden – completed between 1979 and 1981. It covers the sexual thinking of children and has been published in a more technical and academic version elsewhere.[2] Juliette, a sociologist, interviewed all the girls and Ronald, a psychologist, interviewed all the boys, in individual face-to-face interviews using a standardised series of questions.

Our second study, conducted in 1985 and 1986, is the result of a questionnaire to more than 1000 Australian first-year students in tertiary social science courses, asking them to report retrospectively on their childhood and adolescent sexual experiences.[3] This type of study had been conducted in the USA, Canada and England and so we are able to report our Australian findings alongside those from the other countries.[4]

We shall call our first study, covered in Part One of this book, 'What Children Think About Sex' and our second study, reported in Part Two, 'Children's Sexual Experiences'. The evidence given in both is based upon sound statistics and a wide spread of socio-economic and ethnic backgrounds, although the majority of respondents were whites of European descent. While the samples in both studies cannot be called 'national' samples, they are large enough to allow reasonably accurate generalisations about the age groups in the countries from which the subjects were drawn.

The basis for the book then is factual, producing evidence from what children say at varying ages or later as young adults reflecting on their sexual ideas and experiences. Wherever possible we let the young speak for themselves. For example, in looking at 'sexual thinking', specifically about the arrival of a new baby and how it gets out of the mother, we report what a 7-year-old English girl says:

'Is it the ears? (Pause) No, that's a bit silly. It'd get all covered in wax. But I've heard of machines taking things out of ears. (What sort of machines?) Well, the doctor once poked in my ears and got out some wax. Some people have ear-aids. (Pause) It could come out of her bottom, but no that'd be too dirty. (Pause) I think they'd have to cut her tummy open.'

We can see the girl speculating and thinking aloud as she rejects different ideas, then arriving at what she sees as the only possibility.

Here is a more sophisticated description, of 'sexual experiences', from an Australian male tertiary student:

'I remember I played 'Mothers and Fathers' with a female friend. We were both about 9 or 10 years old. Just close physical contact whilst clothed and in bed. It was very pleasurable but not really very sexual.'

We shall see that these kinds of ideas and experiences, far from being rare, are quite common. In the light of what the young report we may have to revise our ideas about what is normal. So much of what children say about sex is regarded as either quaintly funny or condemned as unacceptable behaviour.

The aim of this book is to raise the level of awareness of adults about children's sexuality and to alert them to the positive educational opportunities, as well as the problems, in this sensitive aspect of child development. In so doing we challenge many traditional assumptions made about childhood. It may be that some will find the overall picture a disturbing one. On the other hand, many to whom we have presented these facts in seminars and conferences have found that they make sense and help provide a more meaningful framework for understanding the development of their children.

WHAT THIS BOOK IS NOT

This book is not an apology nor encouragement for the sexual use and abuse of children. Far from justifying the activities of pedophiles, those adults who desire sexual experiences with children, we report how damaging and frightening such sexual encounters can be for children. There is no justification whatever for the sexual abuse of children, for child pornography, nor for the manipulation of children for sexual purposes. All these and related activities interfere with what should be the normal, healthy sexual development of the young.

To emphasise the fact that children are sexual, not only from birth but from the moment of conception, is not to proclaim open house for those who have sexual inadequacies in adult relationships to seek substitute satisfactions with children. Children have the right to be protected from sexual predators, as they have the right to be protected from other physical and psychological threats which endanger their development.

Neither is this book some kind of gospel for encouraging children to be sexually active in the fully matured adult sense before or during their adolescence. We make a clear distinction between adults accepting children's natural sexuality, and encouraging them to be sexually precocious before they are ready or responsible enough. Our advice to the young is to defer such sexual activity until they are capable of a mature relationship based on more important considerations than sex.

In affirming the sexuality of children we are stating an inevitable, natural and inescapable fact of life. Most adults unfortunately pretend this is not so, or they try to minimise its importance in child development. The evidence we produce in this book will, we hope, make the adult world think more positively about children's sexuality rather than negatively and repressively.

Throughout the book we stress what can be done to help children understand both their own and others' sexuality. And in Part Three, 'What Does it all Mean?', we address the practical ways in which we can help both adults and their children come to terms with normal sexuality. We also explore some difficult and unresolved problems and the need for a new theory of childhood sexuality to replace the outworn and inadequate theories of Sigmund Freud.

INTRODUCTION CHILDREN ARE SEXUAL

Many adults assume, because so many remarks made by children appear to be sexually innocent, that they are innocent of sex. Certainly they do say pregnancy is 'a German word for "Be Quiet" ' (English boy, 5 years), or 'It's when you don't smoke or drink' (Australian girl, 7 years). Conception is not only defined as a washing powder, but as 'a fluoride' (English boy, 9 years), 'telling the future' (American girl, 11 years) and even 'It's when you're knocked unconscious' (Australian girl, 10 years).

But the assumption that this widespread misunderstanding of sexual words implies the sexual innocence of children is not supported by the facts. Because many adults resist the fact that children are sexual, we shall review what the experts say on this subject. But first let us define what is meant by 'sex', 'sexual' and other related words.

DEFINITIONS OF SEX, SEXUAL, SEXUALITY AND GENDER

When the words 'sex' and 'sexual' are used, most people interpret them in the narrow sense of reproduction or sexual intercourse. This has been called an adult bedroom definition. If that definition is taken, then it is no wonder that people become alarmed at its application to children and resist the notion that children are sexual.

We have used broader meanings of the words 'sex' and 'sexual' which mean that sex is part of all children's experience from birth. Sex is the physical identity of a person, either male or female. Despite the fact that one 9-year-old boy jokingly said there are three sexes – 'the male sex, the female sex and the insects' – there is in fact a third category. This is the very rare condition of a baby at birth possessing both male and female sex organs, called hermaphroditism. With this exception, sex is a fixed, biologically determined characteristic which gives the individual the body and identity of a male or female. 'Sexual' is the adjective which refers to these physical characteristics, and to the identities and behaviours associated with them. Sexuality involves all that stems from male and female characteristics, and is a broad term covering both sex and gender.

While sex is genetically determined at conception, gender is the social label and connotes the cultural expectations – what is seen as appropriate for males and females. For example, most children in the five countries we investigated think, as do many adults, that females who take up a medical career will be nurses and males will become doctors; or, in business, males will be managers and females will be secretaries. This is what the culture has to date generally expected and may even determine will happen. It will be seen from this that while sex differences are fixed, gender differences can be and are changed as cultural changes occur. Western industrialised societies are making changes in the occupational roles of men and women, through equal opportunity programs, so that male nurses are now more numerous and female doctors quite common; and more women are rising to executive positions in business.

These broader definitions of sex, sexual and sexuality cover not only adult experiences but children's experiences also. From birth children possess a sex, displayed in male or female organs; they are sexual in that they possess and reveal characteristics of their sexual identity; and they are born into a world where sexuality is important. Mothers and fathers, brothers and sisters, aunts and uncles make up their world. Marriage as a sexual, as well as an economic, union is the setting in which they are usually reared. Their early vocabulary has a sexual content and many words and expressions learned in early childhood refer to sexual differences. Sex and sexuality therefore cover a very wide range of children's thinking, experience and behaviour. Reproduction is only one part of this range, developing later when pubertal hormones initiate adult growth.

So what do the experts say about children and sexuality?

THE SEXUAL IDENTITY OF CHILDREN

The sexual identity of a child, whether male or female, is determined at the moment of human procreation when fertilisation occurs by fusion of the sperm from the male and the ovum in the female. Among the chromosomes in each sperm and ovum, there is a special one called a sex chromosome, which can be of two kinds, X and Y. All ova have X chromosomes, but sperm can be X or Y. The chromosomes coming from mother and father combine at the moment of conception to create a female (XX) or a male (XY).

While experts affirm that sexual characteristics are fixed and unchangeable, because they are biologically determined through the sex chromosomes, they can be interfered with or altered by surgery. For example, hermaphrodite babies with male and female sex organs can have one set of sex organs removed surgically. Transvestites and others who wish to have the identity of the other sex may have sex change operations. But these are artificial and usually incomplete interferences with what is natural. Surgery or hormone treatment cannot provide a complete physical change to the sex organs.

For the vast majority, the sexual identity determined at conception remains. All children, however, have to learn in many ways how to be a boy or how to be a girl. In other words, while their sex identity is fixed, they learn the gender roles society expects of a boy and of a girl. Even in these days of unisex, there are cultural differences in how each sex dresses, speaks and behaves. Beginning with the conventional pink for a girl and blue for a boy colour schemes, children are soon introduced to the traditional toys expected for each sex. In the past boys have been expected to be interested in mechanical toys and girls in dolls and domestic pastimes. Parents may not be aware of the often subtle ways they are inducting their newborn baby into gender roles judged to be appropriate by the culture. Parents are powerful and effective educators of their own children in this respect from the very earliest years.[1]

The fact that children have a sexual identity does not mean that they themselves are aware of it in any precise sense. Their first knowledge is certainly not based upon an awareness of their own sexual organ, but rather by the constant references to being a boy or a girl made by parents and other family members. It is not surprising that when we asked 'How can you tell a newly born baby is a boy or a girl?' the replies of young children were of a non-sexual nature.

'If it cries loud it's a boy.'
'If it's got long hair it's a girl.'
'You look at the eyes; if they're blue it's a boy.'
'It's bigger, so it's a boy.'
'The doctor tells you which one it is.'
'If it's got nice clean clothes it's a girl.'

The 5-year-olds who make these comments already reflect some gender stereotypes. But it is also very obvious that many children at this age and even much older are inhibited from mentioning the sexual organs, and when they do they use all kinds of substitute names, because, many assert, the real names (penis and vagina) 'they're dirty. You shouldn't say them.'

Consequently we recorded sixty substitute names for the penis, among them 'pee-pee', 'tinkler', 'tossle', 'weiner', 'hot dog', 'cucumber', 'Joey', 'dildo', 'bird' and 'Gentiles'. There were more than forty words used by children for a vagina, among them 'tooty', 'jobby-wee', 'muffin', 'scooter', 'Virginia', 'Regina', 'Gina' and 'pinky'.

Generally, these substitute names may be classified as words having associations with urination or excreta because of these functions' closeness to the sex organs; analogies; names of people, animals or birds; and anatomical labels. In the early years children are obviously puzzled about why 'I have one and my sister/brother hasn't got one' and few know how their sexual identity is determined. But they are aware of their sexual identity from the first year of life.

THE EARLY SEXUAL ACTIVITY OF BABIES

Some people may be disturbed by the assertion that very young children are sexually active, but if our broader definition of sex and sexuality is accepted it follows naturally that sexual behaviour is observable from the earliest stages of life. Observant parents know that boy babies have erections and that girl babies have vaginal lubrication shortly after birth. X-ray photographs have revealed penile erections of boys in the womb before birth. There are several explanations of this, the primary one being that motions of the body, whether as a fetus or a neonate (a newly born baby) stimulate the activity of the sex glands and lead to physical responses. These responses, of course, are not recognised as sexual by the young and may even go unnoticed or be repressed by embarrassed parents, but they do occur.

Babies also have a basic sexual activity in suckling at mother's breasts, an experience which is a natural part of love-making between adults. While initially this activity is primarily for feeding purposes, it is noticeable that babies sated with their mother's milk will play with the nipples and derive great pleasure from doing so. Sigmund Freud placed great importance on this very earliest stage of development, which he called the 'oral stage', and clearly identified it as sexual in nature. Eating, sucking and kissing, Freud suggests, are obviously pleasurable activities which are part of the sexual development of human beings from the earliest years.

Close skin contacts are not only enjoyed by babies when feeding at the breast but are also part of the sensuous enjoyment of the young at other times. Babies love to be held, to be caressed and to be allowed to explore the bodies of their parents, especially in the early stages with their mouths. Bathtime with its sensuous enjoyment of warm water, fondling and play is a natural form of sexual activity, although many inhibited adults may retreat from such ideas as bordering on incestuous or unhealthy. Yet such sensuous experiences are an important part of an infant's emotional and sexual development.

SEXUAL THINKING AND LANGUAGE AT AN EARLY AGE

Babies perceive their world initially through sucking, tasting and smelling, then by hearing, seeing and touching. Although some of these early sensory experiences are generalised, some of them are quite certainly sexual. Sex differences are gradually perceived through the milky smell and taste of mother, not experienced when the presence of father is felt.

Perception is the raw material of a baby's thoughts, and experts in the last forty years of research in perception have noted that babies are not the passive uninteresting bundles of helplessness they were thought to be. Of particular relevance is the work done at Edinburgh University on the problem-solving ability of young babies.[2] Newborn babies are active learners through the senses, identifying different persons and experiences, and are building up structures of thought from the moment they are born.

Vocabulary generally does not begin to develop in infants until the second year, and language, if defined as 'two words spoken in a meaningful combination', normally begins at about 18 months. But long before this stage is reached babies have served a long listening apprenticeship, learning to identify sounds and to find names for their experiences. This is why parents are advised to talk to their babies, so providing early word stimulation in a concrete manner. Some of the words parents use are in fact sexual words, especially where the baby's body parts are talked about on such occasions as bathing, cleaning and changing nappies. Indeed, early toilet training is a natural setting in which babies learn the names of their sex organs, even if parents use nicknames playfully, such as 'dinky-winky' (penis) or 'pussy-wussy' (vagina). Of course, parents are the most likely origin of the many substitute words for penis and vagina that children frequently use.

Learning to differentiate between the sexes is part of this early learning, with mother, sister, aunts and other females differentiated from father, brother, uncles and other males. The behaviour of the sexes towards each other is perceived, actions of affection and warmth or hostility and coldness are seen. Here are the beginnings of sexual concepts which babies try to under-

Much of this early sexual thinking, and with it the beginning of a sexual vocabulary, is part of generalised social thinking. Mothers and fathers, siblings, other relatives, other babies and infants, tradespeople such as plumbers, bus conductors, supermarket checkers, all crowd the normal child's social world and begin to acquire sexual identities. Some of them also begin to acquire gender labels. The world of early childhood is a sexual world, which slowly develops babies' awareness and contributes to their sexual thinking and language.

THE SEXUAL DEVELOPMENT OF INFANTS

If the young baby has a sexual identity, is sexually active and is a sexual thinker, then these processes are intensified during infancy, the period from about 18 months to about 3 or 4 years of age.

Long before language develops children have become mobile, and they quickly learn to explore not only by crawling and then walking but also by the use of their hands to touch and feel their own bodies. Touching their own sex organs is a natural exploration activity for infants and they soon discover that such touching and fondling gives them pleasurable sensations. Usually such sensations are used for comfort, much as thumb-sucking is, since infants often feel insecure and anxious. This activity has often been named masturbation, wrongly in our view, since the word literally means 'to defile with the hand'. This is an entirely inappropriate expression for an innocent and natural experience, and harsh treatment such as scolding leads to early guilt feelings associated with sex.

Toilet training is another dominant experience at this time and the close proximity of the sex organs to the organs for evacuating fluids and excreta often creates associations of uncleanness which may have a lifelong connection with sexuality. This depends upon how negative, coercive and unpleasant toilet training is. Some parents appear to be unable to control expressions of disgust and anger when cleaning an infant after an 'accident' and so contribute to negative feelings. But parents who are positive, encouraging and accepting during toilet training are those who help their children to retain a healthy view of sexuality because such negative associations are not involved.

Weaning from liquids to solid foods has, of course, been happening earlier and continues with infancy. From being fed, children learn to feed themselves as their hand control improves. Satisfaction of oral needs at the breast or the bottle teat gives way to more sophisticated oral sensations. Some psychoanalysts would maintain that this has a sexual meaning, as all oral activity may have.

During the infancy of many children, a new baby may be expected in the family. Wise parents use such an event as an opportunity to help their children understand what is happening. Even small children can understand what a pregnancy is and where the expected baby is carried by mother. Too frequently, however, parents do not even try to explain what caused the baby in the first place. Neither do they explain what happens at childbirth, by what opening the baby comes out and when. Both of these matters, as we found in our research, are a source of great confusion to children, who resort to all kinds of fantastic inventive explanations in their attempts to understand the processes involved. We shall be reporting in later chapters precisely what these misunderstandings are.

SEXUAL DEVELOPMENT IN MIDDLE CHILDHOOD

These are the years of 4 to about 8, extending from infancy into a more settled period before early pubescent changes begin to occur. It is the time when many begin kindergarten and all begin primary or elementary schooling.

Even before this period children have begun to interact with other children, maybe within their own families, but certainly through the neighbourhood and possibly through informal or formal play groups. This experience with their peers widens children's social horizons but also brings to their attention the differences between boys and girls. Natural curiosity causes many of them to explore the physical characteristics of both sexes and opportunities now exist to make this possible at first hand. As children grow older they begin to play games, many of them of a sexual nature, becoming more and more sophisticated, as we shall see. This is an almost universal activity and both parents and teachers are often perplexed to know how to handle it.

Most parents, and some teachers, at this time, if not before, tend to embark on what is called 'modesty training'. This is the concern, particularly of mothers, to see that their children are dressed 'properly', which obviously involves keeping clean and tidy in appearance, but also concerns the need to keep the sex organs covered most of the time. During babyhood and infancy many parents do not find their young child's nakedness a problem. Then quite suddenly many children find nakedness to be forbidden, and unexplained requirements of modesty are imposed. For many this may be the beginnings of feelings of shame about their bodies, rather than the source of an acceptable reticence about nakedness.

During infancy and middle childhood children do begin to ask questions of a sexual nature, particularly in the period preceding their modesty training – for example, 'What is that?' (pointing to their sexual organ); 'Why haven't you got one like me?' (boy to mother); 'What's it for?' and similar enquiries. Answered in a matter-of-fact way these questions provide an opportunity for helping children understand, as well as acquire an accurate vocabulary. It is sad that so many children believe that correct labels such as 'penis' and 'vagina' are dirty words and invent scores of nicknames to avoid using them.

THE EARLIER SEXUAL MATURING OF CHILDREN

Most people are aware that children are growing up faster; but they are not only becoming larger, taller and stronger, they are actually maturing sexually at an earlier age. World Health Organisation and other surveys show that in Western industrialised countries the average age of a girl at first menstruation is just over 12 years. The average for a boy at first night emission or wet dream and voice-breaking is about 13 years.[3]

Many parents do not know these figures, and for this and other reasons hesitate to prepare their children for what will happen to their bodies, perhaps hoping they will be late developers. In our research we found that girls were especially angry that they had not been prepared to cope with their first menstruation. Equally, boys report being bewildered and confused by first wet dreams.

The problem is not so simple as just recognising 12 or 13 as the usual age of maturing. The fact that the figures are averages means that about 50% of girls will have menstruated in the years *up to* about 12. In Britain research indicates that 2.2% of girls will have menstruated by 10 years of age, 15% by 11 years and 39% by 12 years. But pubertal changes in children which lead up to full reproductive development begin some two years before, as recent manuals on sexual development show.[4] These changes include increases in height and weight, growth of pubic hair, increase in the size of the sex organs and in girls increase in breast size. So to take the British figures, which America and Australia closely follow, about 2% of girls begin these physical changes by 8 years, 15% by 9 years and 39% by 10 years.

The sad fact about these figures is not only that parents seem to be unaware of them, but that where sex education is provided it is usually well into the secondary or high school, by which time most children will have sexually matured. Clearly children have a right to know what is happening to them and what it means, and should not be left unprepared. The evidence is that many children entering adolescence are ridden with serious anxieties, doubts and guilt feelings which affect their later sexual lives.

While it is a relief to know that this earlier maturing trend is perhaps levelling off and that a plateau of development may have been reached, society has been and still is slow in catering for the real needs of children. Childhood is shorter than it was and overt full sexuality which involves reproductive capacity has to be coped with sooner by the young, who generally are inadequately prepared.

What are the reasons for this earlier maturing? Several theories have been advanced. One is that increased and better diets of children have stimulated earlier growth. Another is that society stimulates the sex hormones to develop earlier by much more attention to sexuality being publicly promoted in the media. Yet another, thought to be most valid by experts, is that we are simply reverting to developmental trends seen prior to the Industrial Revolution, when earlier (often teenage) marriages were in evidence, a process disturbed by the move from rural to urban environment and the squalid, cruel conditions in which most children were reared.[5]

THE EARLIER SEXUAL ACTIVITY OF ADOLESCENTS

Because sexual drives are in evidence earlier it is not surprising that sexual activities of a direct nature, as distinct from earlier indirect activities, also occur. Several surveys have been made of these activities which measure a gradation from holding hands, kissing, 'necking' and what is called light petting, through to heavy petting, which may include mutual self-pleasuring (often called 'genital apposition'), incurring pregnancy risks even if actual penetration has not occurred. All these activities are increasing at an earlier age.

The most telling and thought-provoking figures are estimates of age at first sexual intercourse. In 1968 an eminent British researcher estimated that 9% of teenagers had first sexual inter-course before 17 years, but ten years later another researcher estimated it to be 21% by 16 years, and an American survey in 1972 estimated that 23% of American adolescents had first intercourse by 16 years. In New Zealand 25% by 17 years was reported in 1976, and more recent Swedish statistics estimate the median age for first intercourse to have fallen from 19 to 16 years over a period of 40 years.[6]

Since we are dealing with average ages it is well to remember that a fair proportion have this experience before 16. For example, our survey of Australian students revealed that 6% reported the age for first intercourse as being between 11 and 13 years of age and 39% before and up to 16 years. Some 41% had their first full sexual experience between 17 and 19 years.

Now all these are based upon what the subjects in interviews or in questionnaires say happened. While the figures must be accepted with caution, other figures such as those for teenage pregnancies and sexually transmitted diseases in adolescence do generally support this evidence.

It is clear that when these figures of earlier sexual activity are set in the context of earlier physical maturing and delayed or non-existent sex education, then a fairly large proportion of our young are left unprepared for what will happen to them. Ignorance about conception and contraception we found to be common, in teenage girls especially.

INCREASED SEXUAL DANGERS FOR TEENAGERS

Teenage pregnancy rates have been on the increase for a considerable time in many countries, although in some countries such as Australia the figures seem to have levelled off. Even so, the incidence of pregnancy, abortion and ex-nuptial births is still alarmingly high. It was estimated by the Guttmacher Institute in the USA that of two million American girls turning 14 in 1981 about 39% would have at least one pregnancy while still in their teens, and half of these would give birth. The tragic consequences of this were spelled out in a 1986 issue of *Time* magazine in an article called 'Children Having Children'. A British report entitled *Pregnant at School* and reports from New Zealand indicate that the problem has not gone away and in some countries is increasing.[7]

Where sexual activity increases and young people are untutored in contraception, as well as in other aspects of sexuality, the dangers of venereal infection for teenagers are obvious. According to World Health Organisation 1971 figures, syphilis was not increasing among adolescents but gonorrhoea was said to have reached epidemic proportions among the young. Now that herpes and AIDS, for which there are no known cures, have appeared on the scene, infection may be lifelong and in the case of AIDS fatal.

Many respond to these problems by asserting that we must teach the young to abstain and to delay sexual gratification until they find a settled and permanent partner. All sex education programs we have reviewed teach this, but unfortunately the figures show that the provision of sex education by parents is usually inadequate or non-existent, and the provision in schools is usually too little, too late. Sweden is an exception among the countries we researched, since sex education is compulsory in all Swedish schools for all children from the age of 7, when schooling begins. A critical examination of their syllabus shows that the Swedish education authorities have taken seriously the trends we have outlined in this chapter.[8] While there is no proven connection with the provision of sex education, Swedish teenagers show the lowest incidence of teenage pregnancy and venereal disease, compared with the USA, Britain, Australia and New Zealand.

WHY THE NOTION OF CHILDHOOD SEXUALITY IS RESISTED

Sigmund Freud was not the first to perceive and write about the sexuality of children, but he was the first to attract wide public attention on the matter. The assertion of childhood sexuality shocked late nineteenth-century Viennese society and later English society when Freud's work became available in translation. Resistance to the idea was seen among many of Freud's medical colleagues and it is clear that he modified some of his early ideas, particularly on incest, to placate many of his critics.[9]

This is understandable, given the nature of those societies and the attitudes to sex prevalent at the time. Yet even in more enlightened times when sex is more openly discussed and accepted there are hesitations and resistances to the notion that children, as well as adolescents and adults, are basically sexual. A 1981 American symposium on 'Children and Sex' caused a storm in some magazines, where the eminent international authors were accused of being advocates of pederasty, pedophilia and the sexual abuse of children.[10] There appear to be deep-seated fears shared by many in the population to which such campaigns appeal.

Why is it that resistance to childhood sexuality is so strong?

In the first place, much of the resistance is based upon a narrow definition of sex. When sex is thought of solely in bedroom terms, implying sexual intercourse, or solely in reproductive terms, it is natural that adults should react strongly to sexuality in childhood. But given a broader definition, such as we have outlined above, most can accept childhood sexuality as a fact of life.

Much of the resistance to sexuality in children is based upon a genuinely held belief that children should be protected from their sexuality as long as possible. Often the rather sentimental appeal to children's 'innocence' is made, meaning that children are free from sin or moral wrong. There is an assumption that sex itself is sinful or morally wrong and that children should be protected from it. But children's innocence can be maintained in another sense, so that in their formative years they are protected from sexual immoralities which harm their development, such as pornography, prostitution, or depictions of sex in violent or corrupting settings. Certainly children should be protected from child sexual abuse and those who would exploit them for their own sexual purposes. But in order to do this it is not necessary to deny that children are sexual.

An underlying factor which strengthens resistance to children's sexuality is the difficulty adults have about their own sexuality. Fear of sexual rivalry and challenge from each new generation of adolescents is enough to contend with, without having to deal with children. But this threat is more imagined than real, and it will not go away simply by denying that children's sexual identity, sexual activities and sexual thinking exist. The right of children to understand their own sexuality as a normal healthy development should not be threatened by the sexual hang-ups of their elders.

As anthropologists have pointed out, all societies impose sexual limits and taboos upon the young, some harshly and repressively. Most of the evidence from anthropology suggests that the carefree sexual society of natives (the prototype is Rousseau's idea of 'the noble savage') has never existed. Primitive societies in some respects may have been more sexually repressive than some modern societies. Margaret Mead's work suggesting that Pacific Islanders were especially tolerant of pre-pubertal and adolescent sexual activities is increasingly questioned. A classic work dealing with these matters classifies societies as sexually repressive, restrictive, permissive or supportive.[11] Many experts assert that Western societies have ceased to be repressive, are much less restrictive than they were and are slowly moving towards more permissive attitudes. A number of societies are supportive of sexuality in that sexuality is accepted as a normal part of healthy development. On the .other hand, controversy about sex education in schools is indicative of the caution with which many societies deal with childhood sexuality. Even courses in secondary schools are regarded with suspicion in some communities, when it is obvious from the developmental ages we have reviewed that sex education should begin in the primary school.

PART ONE
WHAT CHILDREN
THINK ABOUT SEX

Since children are sexual from birth, it is natural that they soon become aware of sexuality, their own and that of others. In other words, children think about sex from a very early age. Adults are reluctant to admit this, believing sex is something only adults should think about. Yet being sexual with all the physical systems (except the reproductive one) existing and ready to go, children inevitably think about, try to make sense of and find explanations for the sexual world they encounter.

This encounter is probably more frequent and more intense for children now than ever before. Television programs, films, advertisements, magazines and other types of publications deal with sexual matters, continually bringing sex to the attention of children as well as adults. The human body, often with specific anatomical features, differences between men and women, and even sexual relationships, are dealt with, often quite specifically. Soap operas, for example, provide a daily diet of topics such as pregnancy, childbirth, abortion, marriage, divorce, living together, sexual attraction, sexual betrayal and many related happenings. Videos played in the home often contain explicit sexual acts and it is unfortunate but true that children often see them.

The adult world is highly hypocritical in that in so many ways it stimulates the young to think about sex and yet deliberately denies their right to know about sexuality. Many adults even rebuff the natural questions children want to ask, because of their own embarrassments and sexual hang-ups.

Little research exists which tells us what children think about sex, especially in terms of the ages at which they possess accurate knowledge or are capable of understanding sexuality. Consequently, we conducted a survey of what children from

5 to 15 years of age think about sex. Beginning with Australian children, we went on to British, American, Canadian and Swedish children in order to make some international comparisons. We report here our findings from personal interviews with almost a thousand children who discussed with extraordinary frankness the questions we put to them.

Included in this section is how children perceive sex differences, how they think babies are made, how they believe pregnancy and childbirth occur, what they know about sexual intercourse and how their sex is determined, how not to have babies, why we wear clothes and why being naked poses problems. In this section's last chapter (Chapter 7) we review what the children themselves say they want to know about sex, by whom they would prefer to be told and when they feel they should receive sex education.

In view of the basic fact of children's sexuality and the dominant interest in sex seen in the world around them, it is disturbing to report how many childish misconceptions about sex persist. While often amusing, the children's accounts are a sad commentary that we leave them in sexual ignorance for so long.

1
HOW SEX DIFFERENCES ARE PERCEIVED

'How can you tell a newborn baby is a boy or a girl?' we asked
children in our five-country survey of children's sexual
thinking. As well as the answers about length of hair, colour
of eyes, loud or soft crying, and size, other answers are equally
intriguing.

'The nurse knows and tells you 'cause she put the name tag on its wrist'
(Australian girl, 5 years).
'The doctor tells you. He operates on your stomach to see if it's a boy
or a girl' (English girl, 7 years).
'Boys and girls are born differently. Boys come out a different place
[points to navel] and girls here [points to chest]' (American boy, 7
years).

Nothing is more basic than knowing about sexual identity, your
own and other people's. In this chapter we report on what
children know and don't know, first about newborn babies,
then about children growing up into adolescence, then the sex
differences of parents, and finally how they look at their own
sexual identity as a boy or a girl.

NEWBORN BABIES

We have seen how very young children, 4- and 5-year-olds
generally, think about sex differences in terms of physical
characteristics. These ideas, are, of course, erroneous since you
can have big girl babies, boys with abundant hair, girls who
cry loudly and girl as well as boy babies with blue eyes.

'My brother cried like a boy. You could hear him in the next room
he was so loud' (Australian boy, 5 years).
'My sister grew curly hair. It was long girl's hair. That's why they called
her Kate' (English girl, 5 years).
'All big babies are boys.' (Why should that be?) 'Cause they've got to
grow up bigger 'n stronger and look after the girls' (American boy,
5 years).
'Because Mum dressed her in a dress. There's no other way to tell'
(Australian girl, 7 years).

That young children think in these irrelevant physical terms
is all of a piece with their thinking generally at this age. They
make faulty generalisations about the sexual identity of babies
just as they do about many other aspects of their lives. This
is because they seize upon only one aspect of a problem at a
time and so their conclusions are bound to be inaccurate.

Somewhat older children tend to fall back on the word of
authorities, not only what doctors and nurses tell them but what
parents say, because they are authoritative adults.

'My mum told me it was a girl. (How did she know?) The doctor told
her' (English girl, 7 years).

The mystery vanishes with the voice of authority. And as in
most problem-solving at this stage, when asked how the
authorities know children fall back on irrelevant physical details.

'Mom told me it was a boy. (How did she know?) The doctor tells
her. (How does the doctor know?) He looks through a magnifying glass
into their eyes and he tells by the eyebrows' (American boy, 7 years).

Somewhere between the ages of 7 and 9 most children begin
to grasp that babies have quite specific physical features which
are accurate indicators of sexual identity, something which is
common to all boys or all girls. These physical features are not
seen as sexual but rather to do with how water is eliminated
from the body or faeces are evacuated.

'Boys stand up to do the wee-wee and girls don't. (What do you mean?)

Girls sit down. (Why should they do that?) So the pee-pee don't go over the floor' (English girl, 7 years).
'They're different down there. (How do you mean?) Well, some kind of different bottom, the shapes are different. (How are they different?) Dunno really' (Australian boy, 9 years).

Is it that they genuinely don't know, are simply too embarrassed or lack the vocabulary to describe the sex organs accurately? Our analysis of the replies at this age leads us to say it is probably a combination of all three. There is a genuine confusion about exactly what is distinctive about the sex organs of babies (if any distinction is seen at all). There is also recognition of the clear signals many of them receive from adults that this is a taboo topic and that words describing the sex organs should not be used or at least should be heavily disguised.

This is despite the fact that many showed they had plenty of chances to observe the sex organs of newly born babies at bathtime or during the summer at the beach. All the children questioned had one or more siblings younger than themselves and so had grown up with at least one young baby in the family. It is noticeable that Swedish children were more observant at an earlier age and less inhibited when talking about the sex organs.

By the age of 11 most of the English-speaking children had become more observant about the sex organs of babies as the means of identifying them as boys or girls.

'If it's got a penis or not. If it has it's a boy. Girls have a virginia' (English boy, 11 years).

By contrast a Swedish 9-year-old girl says:

'The girl's got a vagina and the boy's got a penis. That's the way it is when they're born.'

Many children know but still display acute embarrassment even when much older:

'Down between your legs where they go to the locker room. It's

7

embarrassing. (Pause) The boy doesn't have a slit down the middle but has a round tube. (What is it called?) Oh, a hamburger and a thing, a penis' (American boy, 13 years).

The evidence is overwhelming that most parents have not used the presence of a new baby in the family to educate their older children in sexual matters. By so doing they have missed an important opportunity to make their children more knowledge-able, and possessed of a better choice of words for describing the sex organs. The exception is Sweden, where sex education has been compulsory in all schools at the primary/elementary level for more than thirty years: parents of the Swedish children interviewed had themselves been through such courses and obviously were able to help their own children at an early age.

SEX DIFFERENCES AT PUBERTY

After the question about newborn babies we followed up with this question, 'Do the bodies of boys and girls grow differently as they grow older?' In this way we were able to judge from the answers whether children before puberty, or in the process of growing through puberty, would have any idea about what was going to happen to or was perhaps actually happening to their bodies. It also helped us to see if and when they under-stood sex differences during childhood and adolescence.

Few younger children had a clue what the question meant or what was going to happen to their bodies, as these replies show.

'They're both the same. (Exactly the same?) No, not exactly the same. Girls have got hearts, boys haven't. Their heart's in the stomach and boys have different bones from girls' (Australian boy, 5 years).

Shades of mother saying 'The way to a man's heart is through his stomach'? Or again:

'Boys are stronger than girls, and can run faster like in the Olympics' (American girl, 7 years).

As in perceiving the differences in boy and girl babies, irrelevant

8

details lead to confusion. Only at a later age do children begin to show a keen awareness, although the inhibitions of sexual language still restrict their descriptions.

'Girls' chests get fat. Boys' still are flat like yours [points to male interviewer]. Boys are stronger and get more muscles' (American boy, 9 years).
'Girls become ladies. (How does that make their bodies different from boys?) Well, they become mothers, they've got to have chests to feed the milk to babies. Men don't' (Australian girl, 9 years).

Occasionally there is an awareness of other secondary sex characteristics, such as the growth of hair, or change in voice, not always accurately observed.

'When people are smaller like me they don't have hairs on their chest. If you have hairs on your chest you're a big strong man. (What about girls?) Girls don't get it on their chest or under their arms' (English boy, 9 years).
'Boys get deeper voices, which sometimes go up and down, like my brother. And they have to shave. Girls don't' (American girl, 11 years).

From 11 on, children make more accurate observations about pubic and facial hair, change of voice, development of breasts, and how the sexes differ in such growth.

'My build will expand, be more sturdy. I'll have hair on my face, chest and groin. My wee-wee erection will start getting bigger. Girls have no hair on their face and chest. Hips expand and they grow breasts. Their bodies will take a different shape. Menstruation happens to girls but I don't know what it means' (English boy, 11 years).

This, incidentally, is the only mention of menstruation by a boy. And few girls before the age of 13 make mention of this rather important body change during puberty, an echo of the lack of preparation they voice later with some bitterness.

It takes some 13 to 15 years before a reasonably accurate description of pubertal changes can be made, such as this succinct account.

'Girls mature earlier than boys and get breasts. Boys mature later and their penis gets bigger and they're generally stronger. They get hairy too. Once a month a girl menstruates and has to wear a sanitary pad. It's a sign she can have children' (Swedish girl, 14 years).

Few from the English-speaking countries are as coherent and knowledgeable as this.

SEX DIFFERENCES OBSERVED IN PARENTS

There is considerable evidence to show that children have great difficulty grasping the fact that mothers and fathers are sexual beings. This is possibly because so much negativism about sex has been spoken, or because sex is unconsciously seen as a nasty forbidden business, that they feel their parents cannot be tainted with it.

Yet this is only one explanation. It may be that since they have grossly inaccurate concepts of their own sexuality, children have considerable difficulties in identifying it in others, especially among those mysterious beings called grown-ups.

In the early years they tend to differentiate mothers from fathers by mainly non-physical characteristics such as the clothes they wear, their haircuts and their rather fixed gender roles. We asked a series of questions about mothers and fathers, how they differed from each other and if the children saw their parents in any sexual roles at all. The most obvious role, the procreation and begetting of children, was rarely mentioned at all, until a series of specific questions on that topic was asked later. We report on the children's responses to this in the next chapter, 'How are Babies Made?'.

Here are some typical categories given by 5- and 7-year-olds showing how they see their mothers and fathers differently.

Mother	Father
She wears spectacles.	He doesn't, only for reading.
Mom's got long hair.	Dad's got short hair.
She's not tall.	He's very tall.
Not as strong as Dad.	He's got a lot of muscle.
Mom stays at home with us.	He likes going for a drink.
Wears skirts and dresses.	Always wears trousers.

Many 7-year-olds and most 9-year-olds think more in terms of the differing family roles of their parents. Few expressed equal or shared roles but usually reflected traditional stereotypes of roles for men and women. Although the questions were asked about mothers and fathers in general, it is evident that most children were talking about their own parents.

'Dad goes out to work. Mum doesn't work, she stays at home. (Does she work at home?) Oh yes, but it's not real hard work. You can stop and watch TV' (English boy, 9 years).

'Mom does the house things like cooking, and washing and making the beds. Dad looks after the car and does repairs to the house. Cuts down the tree branches and that' (American girl, 11 years).

'Mum's quick with figures and helps me with my homework. Dad's hopeless on that, but he does make things for me' (Australian girl, 13 years).

Around 9 years many children refer to certain sexual characteristics of mothers as distinct from fathers.

'Women have to look more beautiful than men. (Why is that so?) Well, to attract men. That's why mothers wear jewellery and make-up. You don't find a man wearing lipstick' (American girl, 9 years).

'Men grow beards and have hairs on their chests. Women have breasts which is so they can have children. (How so?) Well, mothers have to breastfeed babies and fathers don't' (Australian boy, 11 years).

Sex organ differences may be specified directly or indirectly, such as:

'Fathers have Joeys and mothers don't. (What do they have?) Oh they have wimpeys; you know, flat pussies.' (English boy, 13 years).

But this English boy's answer is far from typical. Curiously, at a time when they should be aware of sex differences and are capable of voicing their ideas about them, adolescents become much more self-conscious and inhibited in their replies. In all countries the percentage mentioning the sex differences between their parents actually dropped between 11 and 15. For example the American figures dropped from 60% of 11-year-olds who talked about parents' sex differences, to 39% at 13 years, and to 27% at 15 years.

Other researchers made similar findings among American college students.[1] There are four possible explanations why they are inhibited from seeing their parents as sexual beings. One is the myth, amply demonstrated in our study, of the non-sexuality of older age groups. The old are thought of as 'past it' – sexuality is the province of the young (and by 'old' many teenagers mean anyone over 25 or 30 years of age).

Parents also are regarded as the guardians of sexual purity of the young, enforcing (albeit unsuccessfully) certain rules which inhibit sexual activity, such as being home at a certain time, and rules about dating and going to parties. As rule enforcers they have to be blameless, that is sexless, themselves.

Another explanation may be the inhibition of parents themselves in discussing sexual matters, talking of their own love life, or demonstrating affection in overtly sexual ways such as kissing and cuddling, especially in front of the children.

A more subtle explanation is the awareness of incest taboos in society; within a family sexual limits must be set so that members of the same family are not sexually attracted to each other. What better way of avoiding this than by seeing one's parents as sexless beings? Studies of teenage children of divorced parents show quite clearly that they may be forced to recognise their separated parents' sexuality when parents seek out new partners. This is a source of shock and trauma to adolescents as great as the shock of the divorce itself. In other words, they cannot behave as normal teenagers in denying their parents' sexuality.

It is a strange process that results in children thinking of their parents as the family providers, as the protectors and discipliners of children, and as the loving supporters of their children, but having difficulties in seeing them in their pro-creative role as begetters of children and more particularly the sexual lovers of each other.

CHILDREN'S SEXUAL PREFERENCES

The difficulties children and even teenagers have in recognising sex differences in babies, pubertal adolescents and their parents does not mean they are oblivious to other differences between the sexes. It is one thing to be aware of the fact that men and women are sexually different because fundamentally they have different sex organs, and another to recognise that as a boy or a girl I am different from the other sex. To test out how kids feel about their own identity, and how they see the other sex as different, we asked the single question, 'If you could have chosen, would you have chosen to be a boy or a girl?' They were then asked to give a reason for their choice.

As was to be expected, most children chose their own sex, that is the sex they happened to be. However, a greater proportion of girls than boys 'changed sex' in their choice, evincing a preference for having been born a boy. These reversals are particularly evident around the age of 13, when girls indicate that they are becoming increasingly aware of the restrictions and disadvantages of being a girl.

'I'd be a boy because I'd like to be a doctor' (American girl, 13 years).
'A boy, because then I could go fishing and to football matches with my dad' (Australian girl, 11 years).
'A boy. Because you can stay out late and your parents aren't too scared to let you be out after dark. Boys have it much better' (English girl, 15 years).
'A boy. You can play more sport. Go off hiking on your own, play football, ice hockey, rough games. Girls have to be too well behaved' (Canadian girl, 15 years).
'Boys don't have their monthly periods, having to deal with all that messy business' (Australian girl, 13 years).

Up to 20% of girls voiced these negative sentiments about their own sex, compared with about 5% of boys. Those boys who said they would prefer being a girl did so mainly from curiosity 'to see what it would be like'. Some said 'I wouldn't mind it for a bit, as long as it wasn't permanent, as long as I could change back.' Others said 'It's easier to be a girl', 'You don't get shouted at as much' and 'Girls don't have to get a job or be in the rat race like boys.'

For the vast majority who choose their own sex, the boys express greater satisfaction in the following ways:

'I like being a boy, mucking around. I like jogging, climbing, rugby, soccer, games not normally played by girls. I'm not being a chauvinist pig but I think boys are the stronger sex' (English boy, 11 years).
'Boys have more exciting things to do than girls, like ride motor bikes and camping and mountain climbing. Girls can do that but you wouldn't think too much of her' (Australian boy, 11 years).

An American boy of 15 put it another way:

'Camping is OK for girls but not (lots) of other things. They'd [girls] be tomboys.'

Moreover, boys choose to be boys because they have greater opportunity and wider job choice:

'There's nothing a boy can't be if you've got ability, like the professions or learning a trade, being a schoolteacher or a politician. But if you're a girl all kinds of jobs are closed to you' (English boy, 15 years).

This accepted dominance of males comes out very strikingly in many boys' replies:

'If you're a boy you get perks, the best of everything, the best food. It's natural selection I suppose' (English boy, 15 years).
'I can stay out late and go to the city. If I were a girl I wouldn't have so much freedom' (American boy, 13 years).
'I'm looking forward to being head of a family, that's a man's rightful place, to be looked up to' (Australian boy, 15 years).

These comments may sound somewhat overbearing and egotistical, but that's how the boys see it, as a fact of life.

Girls who are content to be girls do not give recreational reasons as often as boys, often making a virtue of more 'civilised' activities, as does this 7-year-old English girl.

'I do recorder lessons and boys really can't do that. (Why not?) They'd think it cissy.'

Many girls, far from thinking that to be a housewife is to have a life of drudgery, see it as a welcome, less demanding life than the commercial or industrial stress faced by boys.

'It's great to be home and do things in your own time. OK it's a bit hectic round mealtimes but you can go your own pace and relax in the afternoons' (American girl, 11 years).
A girl gets the satisfaction of having children and bringing up a family. Boys are the breadwinners, but that isn't as good as being a mum' (English girl, 13 years).
'I'd stay home and have kids. It's not so complicated as being a man' (American girl, 15 years).

Girls express satisfaction at being girls because they like being feminine. As well as the preference for a more gentle, softer nature, compared with the harsher, more aggressive, demanding male qualities, many girls express delight in taking care of their appearance, making up, and dressing well. Indeed, homemaking and being sexually attractive are the central reasons for girls wanting to be girls, while recreational and vocational preferences and the desire for dominance are the major reasons for boys wanting to be boys. Interestingly, these were trends in all countries surveyed, including Sweden.

We asked a further question of all the children, whether they would choose a boy or a girl as best friend, and why. In the childhood years (5 to 11) their choices were predictably for same-sex friendships, as one can observe in community groups and school playgrounds. To call this a natural homosexual phase of development is misleading and perhaps the term homophilia (friendship for the same sex) is more appropriate. From the age of 13 onwards heterosexual attraction becomes evident for the majority, with girls becoming more interested in the other sex earlier. This reflects the girls' faster rate of physical maturing, and an earlier awareness of relationships as sexual partnerships.

The reasons they give for their preference for same-sex friendships during the childhood years focus on two things, activities and feelings. From 5 to 7 years both sexes wanted friends with whom they could share common interests and activities, such as hobbies or sports. But from 9 onwards right through to 15 for girls, feeling 'at home', relaxed and trusting was the most important aspect. Most boys did not get to the feeling aspect of friendship until 15 years, when, of course, heterosexual relationships are becoming more dominant. Sweden again was an exception, since feelings were the dominant concern in friendship for both Swedish boys and girls from the age of 9 onwards. Perhaps this reflects the human relations work in Swedish schools over the last thirty years.

Examples of the two different reasons can be seen in the following responses:

'Boys. (Why?) Because you can do boys' things like climbing trees and making dens and mucking about' (English boy, 9 years).

'Girls don't play footie [football] and not many play cricket. They prefer dolls and dressing up and such stuff. Boys I prefer. They do more interesting things' (Australian boy, 9 years).

'I like talking to my girl friend. It's good to talk and feel you can share interests like choosing clothes and dressing up. It's real fun' (American girl, 9 years).

'Boys are OK but you need a girl friend you can trust. Not someone who'll blab all over the place. Someone you've got confidence in' (English girl, 11 years).

CHILDREN'S HOSTILITY FOR THE OTHER SEX

In all these discussions with children about sex differences and sex preferences it soon became evident that practically all children made negative comments about the other sex. The comments were not only negative but positively vitriolic in many cases, expressing real hostility.

We were so impressed by the frequency of these remarks that we totalled an aversion score for each child, totting up a point for each negative comment made about the other sex. The results were disturbing as well as illuminating.

What girls think about boys
Boys are rough and dirty.
They're ill-mannered.
Never quiet, always shouting and jumping about.
Dirty messy creatures.
Always chewing with their mouths open.
Show-offs and big mouths.
Yuk!

What boys think about girls
Silly and cissy.
Always want to be clean, they won't get rough.
Interested in clothes, not sport.
They're snobbish.
A bunch of gossips, can't be trusted.
Prissy. You can't be natural with them.
Bitches!

Not many children expressed fewer than five of these or similar remarks, but noticeable among the abstainers were the Swedish children. In the non-Swedish countries the hostile expressions generally increased to a peak at the age of 11, only receding a little at 13 and 15. Girls were significantly more hostile than boys, especially in their teenage years.

Do children in their formative years develop a reservoir of hostility to the other sex? Is it a natural expression of the so-called war between the sexes which continues at a more sophisticated level in the adult years? Or is it acquired by a subtle, and often not so subtle, social indoctrination? While paying lip-service to equality it is evident that our democratic societies still assert in many spoken and unspoken assumptions the superiority of one sex over the other. '*Vive la différence*' may be a joyful expression of sexual differences, each sex complementary to the other, or it can be interpreted as an expression of relief that one's own sex, thankfully, is vastly different from the other. Why has the term the 'opposite' sex become such an established term in our vocabulary? We ourselves never use it, preferring 'the other sex', since opposite signals opposition, and opposition signals enmity.

The evidence in our view shows that sex hostility in childhood, extended into adult relationships making men and women intolerant of each other, is self-inflicted by a society that is only reluctantly beginning to accept sexual equality. What is clearly needed is a conscious effort in family and school in children's formative years to assert both the equality of the sexes in terms of their value and status, and the complementary nature of girls and boys, women and men, in the purpose of human life. The Swedes include in their curriculum what is called androgyny education, which is an attempt to do just this.

So in surveying how children view sex differences from early childhood through to adolescence, we show many different levels of knowledge and ignorance. But even with increasing knowledge, confusions and prejudices abound, from which children need to be released if they are to enjoy happy and fruitful relationships.

WHAT CHILDREN NEED TO KNOW ABOUT SEX DIFFERENCES, AND WHY

The evidence is overwhelming that children from an early age are confused about sex differences, and even when they are older they are inhibited from discussing and correctly naming the sex organs, which are the major distinguishing features of the differences between the sexes.

Rather than discover these facts for themselves, by embarrassing, disturbing and often humiliating experiences, young children can be made familiar from an early age with what distinguishes boys from girls, and men from women. Even before children learn to speak, the correct terms, penis and vagina, should be used for the sex organs. Such terms can be used when bathing or when changing the nappy of a baby, an occasion often watched by other children. Casual mention of what is a girl, what is a boy, can be made during infancy, especially when children's questions begin such as 'What is this?' (pointing to the sex organ) and 'Why hasn't my sister got one?'

Many books for children show quite explicitly the sex organs, with pictures of children and adults. One of these, *What is a*

Girl? What is a Boy? by Stephanie Waxman is an educative way of introducing children to this subject.[2] It shows pictures of naked boys and girls, boys with long hair and girls with short hair, and other features. In simple stages the book reveals what are the essential differences and what are not. Towards the end of the book it states with pictures 'A boy is someone with a penis' and 'A girl is someone with a vagina'. A simple line drawing titled 'Can you finish this drawing?' is provided at the end and children are invited to complete the picture of a boy or a girl.

A parent can do this kind of exercise without the book, but with simple figures drawn on a notepad or a child's blackboard. It can also be done in a simple lesson to a group of children in a pre-school setting or early in primary schooling.

Children also need to know as they approach puberty how these sex differences will continue but develop as they grow. The evidence is very strong that far too many reach adolescence without knowing what changes are occurring or why they happen. This increases their confusion and self-consciousness at a time when they need more assurance and confidence.

We suggest that children from the age of 7 years, certainly no later than 8, be told in what ways they are growing by reference to older children in the family or older classes in schools. Such children grow not only taller and heavier but new features also appear which are the beginnings of growth essential for them to become women and men. This is more developmental than sex education, but characteristics such as the growth of pubic hair, breasts and the sex organs themselves need to be talked about.

We also feel that since the childhood years show increasing hostility between the sexes, home and school should try to close the gap. While the physical differences between the sexes should be known, what both sexes share together also needs greater emphasis. It is a tragedy that many of the hostilities beginning in childhood are projected into adult relationships between women and men.

From about 7 years of age into the teens same-sex preferences tend to be dominant. This has been called by some a natural homosexual stage which society curiously condemns if it occurs among young adults. We prefer to call it a natural homophilic stage (*philia* meaning friendship) which later gives way to heterosexual relationships for most adolescents. It is also curious that if heterosexual interests among older children appear early, adults become nervous and protective, especially of girls. Many adults are content to prolong homophilic groupings among children, that is, to encourage intense same-sex friendships; but if these continue after a certain age they become worried about possible homosexual attachments. Before a certain age they are worried that the young may be precociously heterosexual.

As adults we ourselves need to accept same-sex friendships but at the same time encourage interests and activities across the sexes. If at the same time we have encouraged in our children healthy and responsible attitudes to sexuality, there is little to fear.

2
HOW ARE BABIES MADE?

Young children get quite excited when told the family is going
to have a new baby, although one 7-year-old got it a bit wrong
when informing us his mother was 'inspecting a baby in August'.
Even if there is no family event, most children are sharp-eyed
enough to see pregnant women in the neighbourhood or at the
local supermarket. Many a parent reports embarrassment when
junior draws public attention in a loud voice to the rather over-
weight lady, 'Is that fat lady going to have a baby?'

In our discussions with children we found that once size and
pregnancy are seen to go together they take a leap of logic and
proclaim that all plump ladies are about to give birth. And sometimes the logic goes into reverse, as when a 7-year-old Canadian girl observed:

'She's thin. She's too thin to have a baby. You've got to be very fat
before the doctor lets you have one.'

Even older children get the ideas and the language wrong, as
did one English 11-year-old boy:

'Once a girl is old enough she can get pregnable. (How do you mean?)
Well, it's like a castle that's pregnable. No enemies can get into it.'

After sex differences, how babies originate is perhaps the next
most important sexual understanding children can acquire. The
fact of a pregnancy is not only an exciting piece of news that
can be shared by the whole family, but many modern parents
actively use this time to help children already established in the
family to prepare psychologically for the new arrival.

21

More than forty years ago a researcher in America reported that many children, especially pre-school children, found it difficult to think of a new baby as being inside the mother.[1] This is no longer so. Every child we talked with in our study of children's sexual thinking knew that babies grow inside the mother, even though there is an almost universal belief that it is in the stomach. The big mystery now is not where the baby is being grown, but how it got there in the first place. By the age of 13 most teenagers know there is a separate organ in which the mother carries the baby, but few of them know its proper name, uterus or womb.

How then do children think of the origin of babies? Following an American study in which the investigator pursued the same question,[2] we asked all children we interviewed in five countries, 'How are babies made?' This was varied, if children had difficulties understanding the question, to 'Where is a baby made?' or 'Where does a baby come from in the first place?' Once started on their discussion about babies, practically all children went on many speculative voyages of exploration.

When we compared how the different ages responded it became clear that there is a progression of children's ideas about the origin of babies which can be categorised in six stages. We report the ages at which most children arrive at these stages, although a few well-informed children may get to certain stages earlier and the more ignorant get there much later. What stands out is that most children do not receive adequate information until late in their childhood, but that they provide explanations built upon partial information, hearsay and the gossip of friends. If they don't know they invent explanations of their own in the form of sexual myths. Just as primitive peoples invent myths to explain what they don't understand about the physical world, so children develop their mythologies about sex.

THE GEOGRAPHERS

Preschoolers and children up to the age of 7 tend to think of a place where babies exist, such as 'in heaven' or 'in mummy's tummy'. Further questioning reveals that even if the geographical location is in the stomach babies are not really made but have always been there, pre-existing even the mother.

'The mother always had it there. (Where?) In the tummy, ever since she was a little girl. All girls have them, lots of tiny seeds. Then they grow. (What starts them to grow?) Dunno' (Australian girl, 5 years). 'It was just there. (Where?) Inside the mother, it never was anywhere else. It's just there and the doctor gets it out. (Was it anywhere else before it was inside mother?) No, it was always there' (American boy, 5 years).

The pre-existence of babies for many children may take the form of a religious myth, sometimes associated with the birth of Jesus:

'Babies come from heaven like little stars in the sky. The baby Jesus came from the star. (How do you mean?) The star of Bethlem. They [stars] come down into the mother's mouth when she's asleep. (What happens then?) She swallows it into her tummy and it grows into a baby' (English girl, 7 years).

And a 7-year-old American girl has similar religious ideas:

'God made babies before woman and puts them in girls before they get down to earth. (How do you mean?) Well, they're like little specks, smaller than that [points to speck of dust on the table] and God puts them in girl babies in heaven.'

One can envisage a life cycle of girl babies within girl babies going on for all eternity.

What is noticeable about these geographical ideas is that they are blissfully non-sexual. In a sense, although children do not express it in these terms, all births are virgin births, untainted by any physical or sexual joining. While this is true of the next two stages also, the children's views at this stage are much more theological and timeless.

THE MANUFACTURERS

At about the age of 7 and during the next year or two, children develop the idea that babies are made from materials which are manufactured by God, the medical profession or by fathers. There are even baby factories devoted to this remarkable industry, usually attached to hospitals, since hospitals often have tall chimneys and all factories have chimneys. A neat piece of misleading logic!

'It was made out of bones, then skin, and a bit of hair. (Who made it?) God done it. My mother told me that when other people die God makes them out of their skin' (Australian girl, 7 years).

A more sophisticated theory of medical recycling involves the doctors, a widely held view at this age of which the following is fairly typical:

'They come from dead people in the hospital. (How do you mean?) Well, they've got teeth and bones and skin and the doctors turn them into new babies. (How do they do that?) They put them all together behind the hospital and get them ready to put into mothers' (7-year-old English boy).

Fathers who may have a shed or a workshop in the basement are sometimes seen as manufacturing babies like tiny dolls, although where they get their materials from is something of a mystery.

'His father does it. (How does he do it?) He buys things from the baby shop and puts them together. (What sort of things?) Oh, hair and stuff, and legs. (Pause) I don't know really but he puts them together somehow' (American boy, 7 years).

The manufactured babies face a further difficulty. Since they are artificially made outside the mother, they have somehow to be put into mother's insides. How is this done? Even though tiny, manufactured babies are too big to swallow, so the only feasible answer most children at this stage arrive at is that the doctor cuts the mother open, inserts the baby and stitches her up again. This is the conception by Caesarean we referred to earlier:

'When the baby's ready Mum goes to hospital. (How does she know?) The doctor telephones her and makes an appointment. (Then what happens?) She has an operation. The doctor cuts her stomach and puts it (the baby) in. And that's how it gets in for the baby to be borned' (English boy, 7 years).

THE AGRICULTURALISTS

About this time some children develop an alternative theory. Having heard that babies come from seeds or eggs, children from 7 years on take this literally, which is only natural perhaps, given the assumption that the baby has to get into mother's stomach. Thus the seed or eggs once obtained are swallowed to make the pregnancy possible; an agricultural theory is joined by what is called 'the digestive fallacy'.

'The father does it. (How?) He buys the seed from the seed shop and puts it in her cocoa at night. (What happens then?) She swallows it and it goes down into her tummy and starts to grow' (Australian boy, 7 years).
'The mother eats a lot of eggs. That's baby food. (How do you mean?) It makes babies like lots of eggs and milk. The egg sort of floats in the milk and starts to grow into a baby' (American girl, 9 years).

Some children arrive at this idea earlier, as does this Swedish 5-year-old girl:

'In mother's tummy. I've been there. It's a seed in mother's tummy where she has an apple. No, it's something white, maybe mashed potatoes.'

Seeds, eggs and milk are not the only ingredients that go to make babies. Meat and fish are also seen as essentials by some children, since babies are made into flesh.

'She eats a lot of meat 'n chicken 'n fish and things like that. (Why?)

'Cause the baby's got to have a body, with strong bones. It has to grow big and strong so she eats lots of meat' (Australian girl, 7 years).

Plainly, the food itself becomes the baby since the stomach or tummy is known to be the place where food goes.

Occasionally the seed or the egg, the important source of babies, is not swallowed, but inserted manually, as was cheerfully explained by an Australian 7-year-old boy:

'The father buys the seed. (Where from?) From the seed shop and puts it into the mother. (How does he do that?) He pushes it up her bum with his hand.'

The digestive fallacy involving food or seeds is a step forward in children's sexual thinking because it represents a more biological process. But it is still essentially non-sexual.

Sometimes the agricultural theory gets mixed up with some sexual elements.

'The seed is swallowed into mother's stomach, and sinks into the soil. (What soil?) The soil in her stomach where the seeds is. (Pause) Dad waters it with his thing. (What thing?) You know. His thing, his doodly-do' (English boy, 9 years).

Seeds need watering and what other way, if Dad has a function, than to see him as some kind of gardener watering the seeds in the soil?

THE REPORTERS

Children move from the mythological into a more biological stage between 9 and 11 years, mostly towards 11. These children are aware that something biological has to occur, and most realise there is some kind of physical or sexual joining. But they are vague and uncertain about what it is they report.

'An egg comes out of the man into the mother. (How does it happen?) They rub their belly buttons and her belly button opens and the egg goes in. Doesn't it?' (English girl, 11 years).

'Father has a little dot. When they start to mate he pushes the dot onto her. (How?) He lies on top and the fluid goes inside her. She has a tube connected to the navel. As the baby's coming off, the tube comes out of the navel and the baby is formed' (Australian boy, 11 years).

Others are more informed about sexual joining but there are no concepts about the actual process of fusion between the man's sperm and the woman's ovum or egg. A Swedish boy as young as 5 years knows, yet he doesn't know the details:

'Yes, well they can lay down together and he puts something up her. I can't say what they are doing. It is a pretty ugly word—sexual intercourse.'

In the English-speaking countries most 11-year-olds are just arriving at this kind of reporting:

'By an egg of the man. It turns into a baby inside the mother's stomach. (How does it happen?) It's in his winkle. He puts it in the lady's vagina and it [the egg] goes up into the mother's stomach' (English girl, 11 years).

'A man and a woman. He gets on her and sticks his penis up her slit and the baby starts. (What starts it?) The goo, the wet stuff does it. (How?) Don't know how' (Canadian girl, 11 years).

But some 11-year-olds still express primitive ideas that seeds are passed between parents by kissing on the lips. In this way the seed from the man goes into the woman's mouth, she swallows it into the stomach and the baby begins. This idea is a strange combination of an agricultural theory, the digestive fallacy and miniaturism which is the next stage.

THE MINIATURISTS

By the age of 13 most teenagers have a sexual notion of what occurs in the act of procreation, involving the joining of the sexual organs. But there is one essential feature lacking for a realistic explanation, that is, the complementary role of sperm and egg in the process. There are two kinds of miniaturist, one who sees the baby as a miniature sperm, and the other who sees the baby as a miniature egg.

'The man's penis goes into the girl's vagina and he pushes the seed in the girl and the girl gets pregnant. (How does that happen?) It sort of removes the seed from its spot in a little corner, pushes it out and the spot, that's the seed, grows into a baby' (American boy, 13 years).
'A man and a woman go to sperm. (How do you mean?) The man's cock goes into the woman and the sperm forms the egg. The woman's period makes blood for the baby' (Canadian girl, 11 years).
'It's the little egg in the mother makes the baby. (How does that happen?) The man's sperm it's like a tadpole swims up her thing and hits the egg. That starts the baby growing. (Is the baby in the sperm or the egg or both?) It's in the egg. The sperm just triggers it off' (English girl, 13 years).

Curiously, these children are using the same explanation as biologists in the eighteenth century, before the fusion of egg and ovum were fully understood by scientists. It was called animalculism or ovism. We call it miniaturism because the children see it rather like a tiny photograph of the sperm or egg blown up to full size after a period of incubation by the mother.

It can be seen that the miniaturists also use their ideas to explain how the sex of the baby is determined at conception. This simplistic theory is suggested by an Australian 13-year-old boy, who puts his money on both the sperm and the egg:

'Sometimes it's the sperm that is the tiny baby. If that happens it is a baby boy. But sometimes it is the woman's egg that grows. In that case it's a girl baby.'

THE REALISTS

Even by 15 years of age many kids are still at the reporter or miniaturist stage. But some have a much more realistic grasp of procreation which includes the notion of sexual joining, the passing of sperm from man to woman and the fertilisation process which means the fusion of sperm and ovum into a uniquely new human being. Here is an unusually clear explanation by a Swedish 15-year-old boy.

'A man and a woman have sexual intercourse without contraceptives. There sprouts out sperm from the penis into the vagina. The sperm cell that first reaches the egg fertilises it and then a baby is started. It's either a boy or a girl depending on if it is an X or Y chromosome sperm cell that comes first into the egg.'

An English girl of 13 puts it differently but correctly, including all the relevant features:

'When the man and woman have sex, the sperm from his penis goes into the vagina and fertilises the egg. (What does that mean?) It gets inside and joins it. It forms a cell which then goes into two, then four, then eight and so on and forms a body. It's a kind of black spot with a white ring round it and tiny particles moving inside. It doesn't look like a baby at first.'

There are very few explanations as full or complete as these. Indeed, those who provide a complete picture are in the minority, a rather worrying fact about children at 15 years of age, when most are in their sexual prime and as the figures show are becoming increasingly active sexually.

It may be remarked that a detailed knowledge of procreation is not necessary in order to be a parent. But if, for example, one wants to help teenagers to avoid an unwanted pregnancy, then some accurate knowledge is necessary.

SOME TEENAGE MYTHS ABOUT CONCEPTION

Apart from knowing about contraception as a means of preventing conception most teenagers, including sexually active ones, are under-informed on the subject. Here are some of the myths teenagers have voiced to us.

'It can't happen the first time you do it' (13-year-old active girl).
'You can't get pregnant if your periods haven't begun' (15-year-old active girl).
'It's all right standing up, because the sperm can't travel up the vagina that way' (16-year-old active boy).
'It's OK if you pull out in time' (16-year-old active boy).

All these statements are incorrect. The evidence from many surveys show that teenagers' first experience of sexual intercourse does not usually involve the use of contraceptives. First-time sex does often result in a pregnancy. It is a fallacy that menstruation must precede intercourse if a pregnancy is to occur. As one expert writes, 'In fact, some girls may ovulate even before they menstruate, so that it is entirely possible for a sexually active girl to become pregnant before her first menstruation. Once a girl has ovulated she is therefore fertile.'[3]

Sperm can travel up the vagina to reach the girl's ovum from any position of intercourse. A similar fallacy is often voiced about intercourse from behind. And coitus interruptus is a notoriously unsafe means of avoiding conception simply because seminal fluid containing sperm leaks from the penis before a full ejaculation occurs.

These mistaken beliefs and many others, based upon hearsay and/or ignorance, are fairly widely held among teenagers. It would seem to be of some importance to inform the young of the real process that occurs, if they are to be protected from unwanted results. But our findings are also a serious reminder that most children, and teenagers especially, are dangerously unprepared and therefore unprotected.

THE SEXUAL ROLES OF MEN AND WOMEN IN PROCREATION

Following the questions about how babies are made we asked two further questions, 'Does a mother do anything to start a baby?' and 'Does a father do anything to start a baby?' These were to find out, if they had not voiced it in the previous question, what children know about the sexual roles of men and women in the process of conception.

Younger children (generally 5s and 7s) saw the roles of mothers and fathers as non-sexual and mainly post-conceptual. That is what the children described women and men doing during the pregnancy:

'Mum has to rest and goes on a diet.'
'She's got to eat special foods and drink a lot of milk and baby food.'
'Mom's got to give up smoking and drinking because it harms the baby.'
'She has to visit the doctor and go to the clinic at the hospital every week.'

Father's role also at this age is seen as non-sexual, and supportive of mother once the pregnancy has begun.

'Dad drives the car; makes sure it's working properly to drive Mum to hospital.'
'When she's resting the father looks after the children and cooks the meals.'
'He pays all the bills.'
'He's got to keep her in a good humour when she gets tired and crotchety.'

From the age of 7 to 9 children generally perceive the activities of the two sexes differently. They suggest pre-conceptual activities to help make a baby, but see them as strictly non-sexual (these children are the manufacturers and agriculturalists). Mother

'eats lots of eggs to make the baby';
'stops taking birth control pills';
'takes the pill' (confused notions of the pill actually being a seed);
'swallows the seed in her night drink';
'gets the seed through her belly button';
'gets married'.

31

Father's role is to be the maker or supplier of seeds and the right foods. He

'buys special food for Mum to eat';
'visits the seed shop and buys boy seed or girl seed';
'puts seed in food and drink';
'puts the seed in Mum's bottom with his hand';
'puts the seed in by opening her belly button';
'gets married'.

Awareness of anything like sexual intercourse as an act necessary for conception develops rather late in childhood, as we have seen. And even then, as in the reporter stage, what it is and what actually happens is realised only vaguely. Some younger children make such explanations, but the younger they are the vaguer their ideas become.

'I'm not sure. I think they go to the hospital and ask if they can put their things together and start off a baby' (English boy, 7 years).
'Yes, they get put to sleep by an injection. The doctor puts them together and gets the sperm started' (English girl, 7 years).

Such is the all-powerful medical profession! But others see the mother's role as essentially passive, with father the active sexual partner.

'No, the mother doesn't do anything. It's the father who has to pass the sperm' (Australian girl, 11 years).

Another puts it mainly in the mother's court.

'It's the mother starts it after the willy goes in. It's (the baby) been in the mother all the time but putting the willy in starts it to grow, like water on a plant, the liquid goes in' (English boy, 9 years).

The view of mother as a passive agent is generally held until about 11 years of age, but teenagers begin to report both sexes as contributing sexually, although many are still not sure what it means in detail.

The stages we report in the children's perceptions of their parents' sexual roles in conception are to be found among the Australian, English and American children we questioned. However, Swedish children arrived at these stages much earlier than the English-speaking children, usually providing much fuller explanations at an early age. For example, we found many 7-year-old Swedish children at the reporters stage and many 9-year-olds at the miniaturist or realist stage. This two or more years lead over the other children was an important finding in most of the sexual matters we discussed in our study, perhaps the result of systematic sex education in schools and families over several generations in Sweden.

THE BIG SECRET OF SEXUAL INTERCOURSE

Perhaps the most disturbing feature of the matters we have reported in this chapter is the secrecy about sexual intercourse. Adults do find it embarrassing and for some of them it is impossible to talk about it to children.

Our evidence shows that many parents are inhibited in talking to their own children openly and honestly about sexual intercourse or love-making as the necessary act involved in baby-making. Whilst mothers are among the major sources of sex information to their children they tend to talk mainly about pregnancy itself when having a baby, not how it got in the mother nor, curiously, how the baby can get out at birth. Inhibitions about talking of the sex organs are widespread, not just among children, and such inhibitions obviously restrict the kind of sexual information children receive. Children get their knowledge about sexual intercourse, partial, confusing and often misleading as it is, from playmates, from encyclopedias, radio and TV programs and teachers at school. Perhaps this is why boys seem to know more about sex than girls at an earlier age, since they seem to be less inhibited in their search for to these sources of information.

Why is it that parents are so inhibited? We are products of a tradition of silence and most of us were taught early not to question matters of this kind. As one American boy, aged 11, said:

'It's OK to ask about babies and such, but if I asked about sexual inter-course my father'd really get mad and thrash me. It's just one of those things you never ask about.'

There are some indicators which reveal that these sexual taboos are breaking down and that more parents are less inhibited with their children. But it is a slow process of confidence-building by adults and they often need printed materials and other teaching aids to help them.

Fortunately, there are some excellent picture books available for children from the pre-school years on. The best show in tasteful and accurate pictures what actually does occur,[4] but many books dealing with this topic are so coy as to be useless and downright misleading.

Do children brought up on farms know more than city children, because they see coupling of animals and are often present when foals, kittens, puppies and other young creatures are born? The answer is 'No'. The evidence is that while country children do see the coupling of animals, and even know that this is when they are mating to have baby animals, few of them are informed that this is what humans do. The conscious transfer from animals to humans is not made, since country people suffer from the same sexual inhibitions as city dwellers. The breeding of mice or similar pets, at home or in pre-school, can provide the opportunity for this important transfer of knowledge to occur, but there has to be a conscious effort to do so by adults. Few children will make the inference for them-selves.

The real basis of our inhibitions is an unwillingness to talk not only about the sex organs, naming them correctly and talking about them openly, but explaining what their purposes are. Some parts of the sex organs are for relieving the body of fluids (peeing) but their major purpose, it should be explained, is for making love, enjoying a special closeness and the making of children.

One thing is clear from our discussions – that in many explanations about babies children can be misled and easily confused by the use of analogies. 'Seed' is one example, as we have seen, which causes many children to think in agricultural terms. 'Sperm' rather than 'seeds' can be used without confusion and 'ovum' is better than 'egg', since children think of the brittle, shell-encased hen's or duck's eggs. As one bright 9-year-old girl said, 'Mum has to be very careful when carrying her baby, 'cause the shell might break. (What shell?) The egg shell round the baby. If it cracks or breaks the baby might get hurt and be born too soon.'

But one of the most misleading pieces of information which children are told is that the baby is in Mother's tummy, meaning 'stomach'. This children know is the receptacle of food, and so for the young it encourages the digestive fallacy that babies are formed from special foods and liquids which go down into the stomach. It also leads to gross misunderstanding about what happens during pregnancy, a matter we deal with in our next chapter.

While the geographers, the manufacturers and the agriculturalists provide many charming and amusing accounts of how babies are made, it is sad that so wonderful a process as the beginning of a new life is so crassly misunderstood. Children have the capacity to really understand the process of procreation, from the age of 5 onwards, as the Swedish results convincingly demonstrate, if only they are told the truth.

WHY CHILDREN NEED TO KNOW ABOUT THE ORIGIN OF BABIES

The question may be asked, why not allow children to use their imaginations and develop their delightful mythologies? After all, it is said, childhood is short and children's innocence should be protected as long as possible. Why is it important for children, especially young children, to know about babies in general and the act of sexual intercourse in particular?

First, children need to be treated with honesty, in sexual matters no less than in other areas. Many teenagers have expressed to us their disgust that adults should conceal the truth for so long, especially matters relating to sex. They feel especially betrayed by parents who avoided answering questions, or who have told them downright untruths. No doubt many adults behave from what they themselves perceive to be good motives. They may think the truth will confuse children. Or maybe parents feel they don't know enough themselves to explain conception simply or without embarrassment. What many do not understand is that if there is avoidance of the subject by parents their children will perceive it as dishonesty and the trust that should exist will be undermined.

So when children ask questions about babies, especially at a time when they are excited about a new arrival in the family, they should be answered in honest terms. 'Where does the baby come from?' can be answered in vague terms – 'From God' or 'From the hospital' – which are later seen as dishonest; or quite simple but enlightening explanations can be given.

'Our new baby began by Daddy and me loving each other. (Kissing each other?) Yes, but more than that. You know every boy has a penis and every girl has a vagina. A mummy and daddy put this together and that makes a baby. (How does it make a baby?) Sperm from Daddy's penis goes into my vagina and joins what is called an ovum. Then the baby grows. It's not in my tummy, but a special place called a womb.'

This conversation, reported to us by a mother talking with her 4-year-old son and 6-year-old daughter, led to many more questions.

It is obvious that some of the information given will not be understood by the 4-year-old, but if puzzled a child will come back and ask further questions at a later time. What is established in the conversation between this mother and her children is an honest interchange which builds up trust and reliability.

Second, children need to know about the true origin of babies because the evidence shows how easily they are misled if given partial information or if they are allowed to fantasise on their own. The use of analogies such as 'seeds' and 'eggs' lead to many wrong conclusions, as we have seen. In fact they mislead children into an intellectual cul-de-sac from which it is difficult to get out. Failure to clarify two essential features about babies, that conception comes from sexual joining and that the baby grows in the womb not the stomach, results in considerable confusion. If these two facts are not given, many children's thinking about sexuality becomes retarded by two or more years.

Finally, talking about babies, especially if a new one is expected in the family, provides a setting for children to explore ideas and for parents to tell their children without embarrassment about many features of sexuality which may not arise so naturally at a later time. In the context of a family sharing and seeking to understand the mysteries of life's origins, something of the positive pleasure it all means can be conveyed. The true facts can be associated with warm feelings and positive attitudes, and this is far better than acquiring such information, distorted and often inaccurate, in a sniggering guilt-ridden context behind the bike shed.

3
WHAT HAPPENS IN PREGNANCY AND CHILDBIRTH?

'It takes nine years, I think. (That's a long time isn't it?) Not so long. I'll be nine years old soon and I'll be having a big birthday party. (But isn't it a long time for the mother to have the baby inside her?) Well, she doesn't notice it for the first few years, 'cause it's so tiny. It's only the last year it gets really big.'

This 8-year-old English boy has the numerical unit right but the time unit wrong. And there are even longer pregnancies than this estimated by young children.

Let us first look at these estimates of pregnancy by children, then at how they imagine what goes on inside the mother and finally how they envisage the birth of a baby, particularly where it comes out of the mother's body. Even older children find many aspects of these questions confusing.

HOW LONG IS A PREGNANCY?

The word 'pregnancy' was never used in our questioning because many young children do not know what it means. 'Pregnancy' to many of them may be the name of a restaurant, a railway train or a bookshop. So we asked the question 'How long does a baby take to grow inside the mother?' Even so, some very young children took this question literally and answered 'Three inches' or 'About a foot'. When it was pointed out that it was the length of time we were asking about they quickly switched answers, as this 7-year-old American girl did:

'About nine inches at first, then it grows bigger. (How long a *time* does the baby take to grow?) Oh, it's only a bitty time, about six minutes after the doctor's put it in her tummy. (Why so short a time?) Well, Mom's all ready and warm and when they put it in, they put the baby in, they have to take it out quickly, case it might grow too big. (How do you mean?) It'd be too big to get out if they left it too long.'

In this case, the little girl seriously underestimates the period of a pregnancy. This is so with many children. And she had previously explained that it was a manufactured baby made at the hospital, believing in conception by Caesarean as well as birth by the same method. Clearly she also believes mother acts as a quick pressure cooker.

Or perhaps the analogy is more that of a chicken incubator, the egg literally needing warmth ('Mom's all ready and warm') in order to hatch. Here the baby is inside mother, rather than the mother hen or similar bird sitting on the egg to supply the necessary warmth. While the brief pressure cooker-incubator period is a very common estimate, just as common are the exaggerated estimates of children about the same age. So says a 6-year-old Canadian girl:

'It takes about a hundred years. (Inside the mother?) Yes, it takes a very long time for the seed to grow from a weeny weeny speck. (But that would mean a mother would have to be more than a hundred years old.) Well, the fairies look after that. It's a kind of magic.'

It conjures up pictures of babies born as old as Merlin the Celtic magician, mothers and babies somewhat old before their time.

The older the child the more realistic the estimates of the length of pregnancy become. Girls appear to have more realistic ideas earlier than boys. If one takes 8-10 months as an allowably realistic answer, about 10% of Swedish 5-year-olds achieve this, 3% of English 5-year-olds do, but no North American or Australian 5-year-olds. By 7 years 33% of Swedish children know, 13% of the English and only 7% to 8% of the Australians and North Americans. While two-thirds of Swedish 9-year-olds have got there, only about a third in the other countries have done so. By 13 it is practically 100% in Sweden and North

America but between 10% and 20% in England and Australia are still unrealistic in their estimates.

This illustrates two things. First, that children's concepts of 'time' are gradual in developing, since young children are vague about age, birthdays, clock time and other time-related tasks. They need to be taught these skills. But second, the Swedish results do show how systematic teaching enables realistic time estimates to be made by children from the age of 7. Fantastic guesswork about pregnancy may be amusing, but it does not help a child's grasp of reality.

A curious but natural reasoning occurs with some children, that the length of a pregnancy will vary with the seasons, as does plant growth. A typical expression of this is by a 9-year-old English girl:

'I think it's about six months. I know it's not very long in summer, but it takes a bit longer in the winters. (How much longer?) Oh 'bout 7 months. (Why should it take longer in the winter?) Because it's colder and things take longer to grow in the cold.'

Even 10-year-olds voice this idea of seasonal influence, using variations of light and heat and perhaps moisture to justify different rates of growth.

'Babies take about a year to grow before they're ready to come out. Some take a bit longer. (Why?) Well, it all depends on how much the mother drinks. (How do you mean?) Oh, milk and water 'specially. Seeds have to have a lot of wet stuff to make them grow, and lots of sunshine. Some mums don't drink a lot, some do' (Australian boy, 10 years).

Plants need watering and so do babies, especially at their seed stage. So varied watering will vary the speed of growth. And since children learn early at school that plants can be trained to grow towards the light—the simple mustard and cress seeds experiment—they also know that variations of light will affect the plant's rate of growth. This 8-year-old Canadian boy picks up this idea and puts it succinctly.

'Seven months in summer and eight months in winter. (Why the difference between summer and winter?) 'Cause it's dark in there and things don't grow so fast in the dark. A bit more light gets into the body in summer. (How does that happen?) The mother sits in the garden in the sunshine.'

Time confusion about birthdays is seen in this response of an American boy of 5 years.

'It's nearly two when it's borned. (How's that?) Well, it has one birthday inside when it was made, then another when it came out. We had a nice party when Alice [his baby sister] came home from hospital. (How does that make her two years old?) She's had two birthdays.'

WHAT HAPPENS DURING THE PREGNANCY?

The question 'What happens to the baby while it is inside the mother?' invited the children to provide descriptions of what they think happens during the gestation period. Despite the focus of the question being on the baby, some children still focused on the mother in their replies, giving an insight into some family characteristics.

'Mom's got to drink a lot, so Dad gives her three Martinis every night when he gets back from work. He has some too' (American boy, 9 years).
'No more tennis, says Dad. She's got to stop galloping and drinking' (English girl, 9 years).
'She asks the milkman to come round more often' (Canadian girl, 7 years).

A priceless reply was given by a talkative Australian 9-year-old girl.

'My mother went into training, that's what she called it. She lies on her back with her tummy sticking up and tries to touch her toes. Then she does a lot of sucking. (How do you mean?) She breathes a lot. Then when she's finished, she gets up and has a smoke and says "Let's have a fag. Thank God that's over for the day".'

But most children focus on the baby since they are naturally interested to know what happens to it during pregnancy. As in other aspects of knowing about babies their interpretation may be based on information from mother which is only partially understood or poorly explained. Or they learn by overhearing snatches of conversation, or from their peers. They try to piece all this together into some meaningful pattern based upon the idea that the baby grows inside the mother, whether it takes nine minutes, nine months or nine years.

The idea of a process of gestation, as it is called (from the Latin meaning 'carrying'), is difficult for children, who are literal and concrete in their thinking, because it is internal and invisible, apart from the external symptom of the gradually swelling 'stomach'. Some concrete experience is possible, such as when children are encouraged to feel the fetus moving and kicking or listen to its internal activities. Even so, they are dependent for knowledge and insight about pregnancy upon information conveyed by the adult world, either through verbal or pictorial descriptions. The verbal descriptions may be vague and ambiguously worded. And the pictorial, usually two-dimensional, illustrations can be confusing since some representations of this kind are something of a cognitive puzzle, not really giving children adequate clues. Thus children develop myths about pregnancy just as they do about the making of babies.

From 5 right through to 9 years there is considerable confusion, some of which is caused by the use of the word 'tummy' or 'stomach'. Not only do babies grow out of special baby foods but their growth depends upon getting their fair share of mother's food. Positioned in the stomach they do so directly, as many children indicate.

'The baby eats and eats and eats. (How?) It eats through its mouth, silly. Lots of milkshakes and foods his mum eats. (How does the baby do that?) It comes down her froat tube into her stomach and it [the baby] opens its mouth and swallows it. (Does anything else happen?) No, the baby's got nothing else to do 'cept eat so it can get big' (English boy, 5 years).

The same idea with some quite imaginative embellishments

is expressed by an American 7-year-old girl:

'It sits in the dark and waits for Mom's mealtimes. Then she (mother) eats a lot of good food like milk and eggs and butter, and the baby catches as much of it as it can and eats some of it up. (Only some of it?) Yes, the mother has to keep fed too, but the baby takes most of it. (Does the baby prefer any kind of food?) Well, all the soft food, like spaghetti and jelly 'cause it's got no teeth. Stuff like steaks and potatoes are no good, unless it's mashed potatoes.'

Here the idea of a separator is implicit in that both mother and fetus have to be fed. Most children questioned about this fail to come up with any satisfactory mechanism.

Some children from about 10 years onward do begin to think otherwise, as does this English 11-year-old boy.

'I think women must have two stomachs. (Why?) 'Cause the food mother eats would slosh all over the baby. No, it's a separate kind of bag and it's fed by a tube. (What sort of tube?) It's a food and breathing tube to its mouth. (Where is the other end of the tube?) It's fixed to the mother's belly button, from when *she* was a baby.

Just the reverse of reality; the umbilical cord is fixed to the baby's navel.

However, eating is not the only activity which goes on inside mother.

'Well, you don't see what goes on in there, but I think it lies on its back and stretches. That's how it kicks. It's got to keep doing exercises in there so it'll be OK when it comes out to be borned' (Australian girl, 7 years).
'All that kicking and stuff it's very tiring. So the baby has to sleep a lot. When it gets bored it watches TV. (How does it do that?) Through a little hole, through the belly button thing' (Swedish boy, 5 years).

Let's hope he has a remote control to choose the right program!
When not eating, kicking, resting or watching TV, babies have other activities, particularly calling attention to themselves.

'It cries and cries in there, but no one can hear it. It's sinsulated in the stomach. It's the only way it can try to breathe, by crying and yelling and fighting for its life' (American boy, 9 years).

How the baby breathes is a source of concern to many young children since they cannot conceive of an organism without the need to eat or breathe. A long speculative question comes from an Australian girl of nearly 8 years.

'I'd like to know how that baby breathes. I mean, it's in danger of suffocating isn't it? It's got to get some air somehow. Maybe it's got a special tube to the outside. We've got air conditioning at home.'

The last sentence may be an afterthought, or perhaps it is the hint of a mechanistic explanation.

Other children resort to religious explanations about how a baby grows or survives for the period of a pregnancy.

'There's no air opening and it has to breathe. It'd just die in there after a few minutes. (What happens?) Some do die but God looks after most of them and they're all right. (What does God do?) It's magic. He breathes on them, blows special air in to keep it fresh air' (English boy, 7 years).
'It just grows and grows. (How does that happen?) God does it. He's in charge of all little babies. He takes care of them, makes sure they're warm and cosy in there. He [God] stops his mum having a fright and sees she doesn't smoke or drink' (American girl, 6 years).

Older children are not preoccupied with what are in fact largely irrelevant details, and begin to envisage growth as a gradual development from something formless into a human body. The concept of gradualism or evolutionary growth is implicit in many of the statements made by children of a wide age range.

'The baby grows. I've seen disgusting pictures where the feet and hands are like buns' (Swedish girl, 7 years).
'It grows with mother's energy, or God's, I don't know. First they're little round balls, then their legs and bodies grow, and their heads' (English boy, 7 years, estimating length of pregnancy to be four years.).

'I saw this picture of a baby. It floats in a sort of water, and swims around. That's why I'm a good swimmer' (Australian boy, 5 years).
'It's in a kinda plastic bag and looks like a little monkey at first with a big head. If it's born too early I suppose it is a monkey' (American boy, 9 years).
'It gets more prepared to go into the outside world. It gets a head, a face, then arms, legs, body and its insides. It gets hair and teeth and eyes' (Australian girl, 9 years).

As children grow older their ideas of gradualism become more explicit, with some biological inaccuracies, but still involving a prehuman organism developing into a fully human one.

'It grows a tail like a fish and feeds through the mother's fallopian tube. The tail disappears as it grows, and begins to look like a baby' (English boy, 9 years).
'It's like a little animal after it's a blob. Then a fish and then it's a baby, not as it comes out but with a bigger head. The rest of the body catches up. It takes about ten months' (Canadian boy, 11 years).

The more sophisticated descriptions still contain some errors but a systematic theory of development from embryo to baby can be seen.

'The cells join and make an embryo, a big cell or a lot of cells. These produce more cells and some eggs, and grows head and brain and eyes. It gets nerves which grow. It just goes on like that because of the cells' (Australian boy, 13 years).

This evolutionary cellular development also contains a more accurate idea of how the baby gets its energy or 'food' for growing.

'It's the nutrients it gets from the mother's blood' (English boy, 15 years).
'It's connected to the mother by the placenta, which protects it and gives it oxygen and makes it grow. It develops its own characteristics. It all happens in the womb by meiosis. It takes three months before it looks like a baby' (Australian girl, 15 years).

Such descriptions are a long way from the simplistic ideas of this 11-year-old –

'The baby's got to be a fish first with a tail. I'm glad it dropped off before I was born.'

– or this 9-year-old

'My dad told me I looked like a tadpole at first. That's before I was born. So I've always had a small head.'

Sometimes they get it nearly right, using the correct words but not knowing what the words mean. The internal tubes also are somewhat confusing, being sometimes mistaken for the umbilical cord. The placenta is the organ which grows in a woman's womb and to which the embryo, and later the fetus, is attached by the umbilical cord. Oxygen and nutrition from the mother is filtered through the placenta to the baby and waste products are returned to the mother the same way. So, this Canadian 11-year-old gets some of it right, as we see:

'The placenta grows to feed the baby. (What's the placenta?) It's a kind of bag which covers the baby to protect it [she means the amniotic sac]. It gets blood from it so it can live. The umbilical cord finds the baby. (How?) Through its belly button from the food in the mother's blood.'

Even the most senior students have difficulties knowing all these kinds of details, because the whole process is invisible. This topic, however, causes nothing like the difficulties revealed in the answer to the question 'How does a baby get out of its mother's body?'

HOW ARE BABIES BORN?

It still is a big mystery to children how babies are born. Questioning of a few children prior to our study showed that they are plainly puzzled by two vital matters, where the baby gets out, and what starts the process of childbirth off at the right time. A few younger American children thought the right time, naturally, to be Labor Day, but others thought that a festival such as Christmas Day, associated with the arrival of the baby Jesus, was more appropriate. Although Mum may have said 'We are getting a new baby around Christmas time' this easily becomes translated as 'for Christmas' with all the other cellophane-wrapped goodies around the Christmas tree.

To find out the extent of their confusion and what they actually did know we asked all the children two basic questions. One was 'Where does the baby get out of the mother's body?' and the other was 'What makes the baby get out at . . .?' (citing the estimated time of pregnancy they had given).

Up to and including age 11 practically all children, except in Sweden, had difficulties in answering both questions. A few of our children had actually been present at the birth of their baby sibling and so could answer the first question quite accurately, although the second question was a puzzle to them also. For most children, despite a more open approach there is obviously still so much secrecy attached to childbirth that they have to use whatever their minds or imaginations have to work on, or simply guess the answer.

WHERE DOES THE BABY GET OUT?

The truth is, unless you actually know (and even when you have been told, it may seem too incredible to believe) there does not seem to be a suitable aperture in a mother's body through which a child may be born. We heard from the children about every possible opening, some discussed at length and one by one rejected as impossible. A few possible openings were recognised as already blocked, such as the eyes – 'there's eyeballs getting in the way' – and the ears – 'Oh, too much wax.' How on earth can a baby the size of a new arrival really squeeze through some of the gaps in the human physique?

Many children in middle childhood find no aperture possible and so arrive at the very logical conclusion that the only way is to cut the mother open. Official statistics state that in the UK the percentage of births by Caesarean section is no more than

10%, in Australia about 15% and in the USA about 18%. Yet many children put it at 100%!

However, for the very youngest the problem simply does not exist because they are fixated on the word 'delivery' which conjures up some outside parcel delivery agency. Ignoring the baby being in the body, which they know, they still give such replies as

'Santa delivers the baby at Christmas, like the baby Jesus' (Canadian girl, 5 years).
'There's a delivery van comes up with boxes and parcels and stuff. The driver delivers the babies that way' (English boy, 5 years).
'My Mom says there's a delivery room at the hospital. (Why is it called that?) It's where you pick up the baby when it's ready' (American boy, 7 years).
'The doctor delivers the baby. (How does he do that?) He gets it from the hospital workshop and brings it into the ward and gives it to the mothers' (Australian girl, 7 years).

The delivery business appears to be serviced also by nurses, clergymen, policemen and even gardeners, whose associations with seeds plainly qualify them to deliver the required goods. A few fathers may 'deliver' in this way, but most are too busy with the wife, the other children or housework to be involved.

Most children are simply very puzzled and express their puzzlement in various ways:

'It's got to get out somewhere, hasn't it? (Certainly, but where?) Oh, maybe the nose. Some people have big noses. When Mom breathes real hard it comes out there, I think. It's all to do with tubes and things' (American boy, 5 years).
'It comes out of the mouth. They operate by a special machine. Is it a stomach pump? I once saw baby crocodiles on TV in the [crocodile] mother's mouth. Well, it's in the stomach, it's natural it comes out of the mouth. That's where the mother swallowed it when it was tiny' (Australian boy, 9 years).

No doubt for all these cases they bring in the ear, nose and throat specialists! Fantastic as these speculations appear, they are widely held among 5- to 9-year-olds who have been given no explanation of where the birth canal is. Some, such as this 8-year-old girl, use a kind of mental check list and reject each idea in turn. Her reasoning is speculative and charming:

'There's no obvious place is there? I mean, the eyes are already full, it couldn't squeeze past. Ears? No, that's silly, not big enough. The nose? (Laughs) It'd be a bit of a narrow squeeze. (Giggles) Funny if you sneezed and the baby blew out . . .' (Canadian girl, 8 years).

She is one who finally settles for the Caesarean theory since there are no satisfactory alternative openings wide enough for a baby to emerge.

A small but still sizeable group of children had one possible convincing variation. Because they know that the navel is somehow involved in birth, they think of it as a small hole temporarily blocked but opening for childbirth. Some actually call it a birth button and its closeness to the belly, i.e. the stomach, makes it appear a feasible proposition. In fact many children aged between 7 and 9 and even a few 11-year-olds believe that sexual joining is when the man's and the woman's navels come together. If the man's seed goes through his belly button into that of the woman, what is wrong in thinking the reverse happens, that the baby comes out of the mother's, during childbirth? Here are some examples.

'The belly button. It's the birthday button where you was born. (How do you mean?) Everyone's got one. It's where you come out of your mother's tummy. It's where my baby will come out when I have one. (Don't boys have them too?) Yes, but they don't have babies. It's where they're joined to their mum's belly button. It's where they come out too' (English girl, 7 years).
'Is it the button? The umbilicus button? It's where the goo came through from the father into mom's stomach. It's a small opening in the tum. When the baby's born it turns with its head pointing to the button. Then (pause) the button opens up. I think the doc stretches it open, has to cut it sometimes. The baby comes out head first. That's why it has to lie that way' (Swedish boy, 9 years).

'It comes out where the birth button is. It used to be a hole but it's kinda shrivelled up when it's not being used. They stretch it with exercises and things before the baby is born' (American boy, 9 years).

Talk about navel encounters! But it does all make a kind of sense to immature minds seeking to formulate a coherent theory of childbirth.

For older children the more realistic theory of how babies get out stems from a vague knowledge that it all happens some-where below the hips. These children talk of babies being born between the legs, but unfortunately the kids confuse terms like 'bum', 'bottom' and 'fanny', not realising that in the female there are three openings in this region. There is the vulva and internally it's the vagina, not only used for sexual joining but also providing the birth canal or exit during a normal birth (children frequently refer to this as the 'hole', the 'virginia', the 'crutch', the 'hamburger', the 'pussy' and by many other expres-sions). Then there is the urethra a woman uses for evacuating fluids; this is referred to severally as the 'pee hole', the 'wee hole' the 'dinky', 'doo-doo' and many other variations. Third, there is the anus, used for evacuating solids or the faeces; children refer to this aperture as the 'poohole', the 'shit hole', 'arse' or 'arsehole', even 'fanny' and 'that place, you know'.

Of these three openings it is the anus which provides the birth exit in the speculative thinking of many children up to the age of 9, even up to 11 years of age. Twenty per cent of Americans aged 11 still believed the anal canal to be the only birth exit possible. We don't need to search far for the reasoning behind this belief. Since a large number believe babies are made by mother eating special foods, if food comes out of the anus, so do the babies which are made and grow from the special baby foods mother consumes.

'It comes out of the bum. (What's the bum?) A special part of the bottom, where you get rid of poo. It's big enough if you try hard enough' (English boy, 7 years).
'It comes out of her bottom. (How do you mean?) It's the only place it can come out of, 'cause it can expand, like when you go to the toilet. It's sometimes hard to get it out, but if you're patient it will come. (What

will?) Your poo. I suppose Mom must take something to help the baby just like when you're consummated [constipated]' (Canadian girl, 9 years).
'The fanny is where it's born. (Where's that?) Out of her bottom, at back, between her legs. I've seen pictures of it. (Can you tell me a little more?) It's kinda embarrassing, but it's where you get rid of shit' (American boy, 9 years).

One Australian, a 9-year-old boy, elaborates on what we have called 'the digestive' explanation. After identifying the anus as the birth canal, he goes on to provide a detailed system which justifies his mistaken ideas.

'A baby's made out of all that milk 'n eggs and stuff, all that baby food. Well, it's gotta be digested, right? When it's made into a baby it comes out with the waste food. There's no other way. It's gotta be the bum.'

All these misunderstandings seem to originate, as we have observed already, from the baby being thought of as in the stomach. In addition some children do not know about sexual intercourse, or if they do they don't associate it, as some primitive peoples do not, with conception. So the digestive food fallacy is as good an explanation as any for how children are born, and the anus is the only possible birth exit.

An operation by which a small percentage of babies are born is when the baby is removed from the womb by cutting through the abdominal and uterine walls. The name normally given to it is a Caesarean (or Caesarean section), so-called because Julius Caesar is said to have been born this way. Another name is hysterotomy, and it is necessary when delivery cannot take place normally through the birth canal of the vagina. Kids often know about this operation from overhearing adult conversations. So, in perceiving no opening large enough to serve as a baby's exit, it is natural many kids should think of the Caesarean section, not as an emergency method, but as the normal method of childbirth. Our interviews revealed that a large number of those aged between 7 and 11 years in several countries believed this to be so. Here are some typical examples:

'She goes to hospital to have it. (What happens there?) The doc puts her on the operating table and cuts open her belly. They lift the baby out and it's borned. (Why do they need an operation?) 'Cause it's the only place it can get out. All the babies are born that way' (American boy, 9 years).

'The doctor uses the scalpel and cuts her open . . . (Why is an operation necessary?) The holes around the bottom are too small. (Is that so for all babies?) Yes, nearly all of them. That's why they have to go to hospital' (Australian girl, 10 years).

'It's in the operating theatre. (Why is an operation needed?) 'Cause there's no other way. They stitch mom up afterwards and it soon heals. I saw it in 'General Hospital' on TV. It's called a Caeseran' (English boy, 11 years).

Many of the younger children see a slightly more complete picture, based on the theory that a baby must come out of the same opening it went in. For them mother has to be opened up in the first place, so why not a second time?

'The doctor cuts mom's stomach open and takes the baby out. It's where they put the baby in, the first time. They take out the stitches and the baby just comes out' (American girl, 7 years).

What can be neater than that? Zip open the stomach, put the baby in until incubated to the right size, then zip open once more for delivery – conception *and* childbirth by Caesarean.

WHAT CAUSES CHILDBIRTH AT A PARTICULAR TIME?

Our second question after 'Where does a baby get out?' was 'What makes the baby get out at . . .?' (citing the estimated time of pregnancy they had given, from six minutes to six years). Childbirth is composed of three stages – labour, delivery and the afterbirth. Few children know of the third stage, and the first two stages of labour and delivery are understood only partially, right up to the age of 13 years. This question was really focused upon what starts the labour.

The young have the strangest notions about this. As one 5-year-old Australian boy said:

'It gets so hot in there, he [the baby] has to get out to have a drink.'

And a little English girl of 7 years says:

'The baby's all crunched up inside there. It stretches and then starts kicking its way out.'

And another 7-year-old, an American boy, says:

'It's starving. It's fed up with milk and stuff and wants some proper food. It can't get enough inside.'

Then there's the tedium of it all, especially if it takes a few years and you can't watch TV through mother's belly button:

'After a time it [baby] gets tired of sleeping. There's nothing to do, and it's all dark. It has to get out for a change.'

Most children see babies having the initiative. The baby decides for reasons of thirst, hunger, freedom of movement or sheer boredom that the time has come, then terminates the pregnancy by various activities. The baby crawls up the tunnel, or kicks its way out, or squeezes past the blockages in the nose, throat or anus, and forces an exit, or shouts to the doctors to cut the stomach open.

'After all that time,' says one cheerful 6-year-old, 'everyone is inspecting it!' And an Australian 7-year-old boy, obviously a fervent educator, says:

'It has to get out to see the world, to see his mother and family. (How do you mean?) So it can learn to live. So it can learn to write and learn how not to spill things over the carpet.'

Older children do begin to perceive that it's not the baby's initiative that begins childbirth but some physical necessity felt by the mother. Sometimes it is expressed in crude terms that it must happen to save the mother:

'She [the mother] might just burst wide open if the baby gets too big. It can't go on growing for ever and ever. Anyway, the mom wouldn't be able to stand up without falling over on her face' (American girl, 11 years).

This is a long way from the 15-year-old English girl who perceives:

'It's a big bubble and it might break. The waters in the sac break. The baby is fully formed, it's ready to live on its own away from mother. It's got all its organs and is ready to breathe.'

Yet those much younger who've heard vaguely about a bubble breaking often get it somewhat confused, again putting the initiative in Baby's court.

'There's this bubble like a balloon and the baby's inside it. When it's ready the baby makes a hole in it and gets out. (How does it do that?) By kicking. Maybe someone pricks it with a pin' (Canadian boy, 7 years).

Obviously a little 6-year-old saw in the magic word 'labour', whispered among the nurses at the clinic, an association other than the Labour Day holiday. She simply announced that when the new baby was about to appear 'they had to get a labourer'. And another misheard the need for mother to have contractions before father could take her to hospital, as 'My mom's contradictions started at three o'clock in the morning'.

Some children absorb misleading facts from TV shows or from conversations overheard and state that 'Most babies are born in taxis.' We enquired of one 8-year-old Australian why he'd said this. 'My brother,' he said, 'was born in a taxi just outside the hospital!' – a neat example of reasoning from one particular event to a general law.

One English girl aged 9 described what she had heard from downstairs while a lot of mysterious activities went on upstairs.

'When they thought the baby was coming, the doctor sent down for a lot of hot water. (What do you think that was for?) So he [the doctor] could wash his hands I suppose, or maybe make some tea.'

And another 9-year-old, an American boy, was among several we interviewed who had actually witnessed his baby sister's birth in the hospital. Almost bursting with pride, he told us what an amazing thing it was to see happen.

'It was great. We saw it all happen, little Mary coming out head first. My brother and me stayed to see it all, but Dad had to go into the corridor and be sick.'

Describing childbirth, one 11-year-old Canadian girl said it was important to have a midwife there. 'What's a midwife?' we enquired. 'Oh, that's a wife who hasn't got married yet.' But the prize for mispronouncing a vital part of childbirth goes to the 11-year-old Australian who solemnly stated that after a successful childbirth you had to 'cut the Young Billy Cord'.

Swedish children generally could describe the process of childbirth including the need to recover the afterbirth, which none of their English-speaking cousins knew about. All children, however, did know about some of the things that had to be done to the baby immediately following birth:

'The baby has to be slapped, because it's crying too loud' (American boy, 7 years).
'Once it's come out it has to be washed 'cause he's not been to the loo [bathroom]' (Australian girl, 8 years).
'The nurse clears out its nose. (Why does she do that?) Babies don't have handkerchieves' (English girl, 11 years).
'The mother holds the baby in her arms and the baby nests in her breasts' (English boy, 5 years).

So many of these misunderstandings and confusions could be overcome if two facts were simply stated. First, the baby comes out through the mother's vagina. It is, of course, necessary to explain what the vagina is for in the making of babies, and that behind it is the womb or uterus in which the baby grows – definitely not the tummy, the belly or the stomach. Second, that the opening of the vagina, although narrow, expands wide enough for a baby to come out. There are several tastefully drawn picture books which show this process at work, books suitable for both pre-school and primary (elementary) school children. A visual version is far more effective than fumbling words.[1] There is the growing practice of allowing children to watch (if the birth is likely to be without complications) the arrival of the new baby brother or sister. Not everyone is willing to accept such a practice as appropriate for their family, but where it does occur it is worth months of sex education by talks and pictures. First-hand experience is the greatest teacher of all.

Parents and teachers should take care to stress that an operation (the Caesarean section) is only needed in an emergency. Otherwise girls in particular may begin to have frightening negative feelings about the necessity of being cut open, if they want to have babies.

WHAT CHILDREN NEED TO KNOW ABOUT PREGNANCY AND CHILDBIRTH, AND WHY

Children are naturally curious about what is happening around them. If we are sensible parents and alert teachers we try to satisfy their intellectual curiosity when it arises, since this is the best way children learn. Young children appear to learn very effectively long before they arrive at school, by their normal inquisitiveness. This spirit of enquiry, of wanting to know, includes the family, especially any new arrival. And even if a new baby is not expected in their own families, children usually know of households where a new baby is expected. All around them, in the streets, in supermarkets, at school gates waiting for their children, pregnant women are visible.

Yet some parents, presented with a golden opportunity to enlighten their children, either withhold important information about pregnancy or talk to their children in vague generalities. Either way their children remain confused or begin to formulate those mythologies which only retard their thinking and delay understanding one of the most fascinating and enjoyable experiences of their lives.

It is true that they have no immediate use for knowing about pregnancy and childbirth, since it will be some time before they are potential parents themselves. But why should we delay when a few words of simple explanation can obviate years of perplexity and confusion? In most other areas of learning we build up knowledge slowly, as in number activities simple sorting and counting precede arithmetic. Children need to be introduced to simple ideas early so they can digest and make sense of them. And where sexual matters are concerned, experience shows they need to be told many times before they can sensibly grasp what it all means.

So where pregnancy is concerned there are two basic ideas which need to be known by even very young children. First, when a woman is pregnant, the growing baby is not in her stomach but in a special place called a uterus or a womb. If this is established there is less confusion about the food the mother swallows and ideas such as 'the digestive fallacy' may be avoided. Second, it can be clearly stated that a pregnancy takes about nine months. Several books contain a pictorial pregnancy calendar, designed for children to see how long each stage of pregnancy takes and how the baby grows in complexity. Peter Mayle's book *Where Did I Come From?* is especially clear.

The three basic facts, the womb, the nine-month pregnancy and the birth exit, should also be repeated during later childhood and in the pubertal years. More complex details can be added for older children, but unless the basics are grasped even older children will tend to get it all wrong.

4
SEXUAL INTERCOURSE AND SEX DETERMINATION

These two areas are closely linked to the previous questions about how children perceive sex differences in men and women, how babies are made and what happens during pregnancy and childbirth. We have already seen that sexual intercourse is a big mystery to children or so embarrassing a topic that many children hesitate to discuss it. And children are very vague about what determines a child's sexual identity as a boy or girl at the moment of conception. On both these questions the following statements are quite typical.

'Dad gets on top of Mom, I think, and they do a lot of loving. (What happens?) I don't really know but I've heard them at it, they make a lot of noise, 'cause their bedroom is next to mine. (What did you hear?) At first I thought they were having a fight. (Pause) He puts his thingo in her belly button and a lot of jelly goes in, I think' (American boy, 11 years).
'The egg and the squirm when they meet, kind of fight it out. The bossier one wins. If the egg wins, it's a girl. If the squirm wins it's a boy' (Australian girl, 11 years).

The American boy is so vague he does not connect the love-making he describes with the making of babies. The Australian girl does make the connection but gets it amusingly wrong. Since we asked some further questions on these two matters we shall report on them in this chapter.

SEXUAL INTERCOURSE

In our first trial interviews it was apparent that children are aware, however vaguely, that some kind of special activity of an intimate nature goes on between men and women. From about 11 years of age children referred to sexual intercourse by many pseudonyms such as 'having it off' or 'doing it' or more specifically humping, rooting, having contraceptions, poking, bagging, rogering, pumping, knocking, rolling in the clover and many others. With increasing age children began to see such activity as necessary for the conception of a baby.

By 9 years 100% of Swedish children could talk about sexual intercourse as could 48% of English, 40% of Australian and 17% of North American children in our sample. By 11 years the figures had become 95% for Australians, 80% for English and 50% for North American children. By 13 years practically all children in all countries talked about and named in some way the act of sexual intercourse, although some 6% of North American 13-year-olds were either ignorant or reticent about the topic. Some may express surprise that the North American children seem so inhibited. Certainly, in many ways the USA is a very sexually aware society, but it is far from being everywhere sexually enlightened. Indeed in that country can be found the fiercest antagonisms to sex education, which is condemned by many powerful minority groups as a corrupting and pornographic influence upon children. In our experience the North Americans are the most ignorant sexually.

Towards the end of the interview, where and only where children had made some reference to sexual intercourse by name or nickname, we asked a further question, 'Apart from wanting a baby why do people want to . . .?' (have sex, intercourse, screw, etc.), using the precise words used by each child. Only 13% of the Swedish children saw no other reason, whereas about 50% of children in the English-speaking countries saw having babies as the sole reason for sexual intercourse.

'It's just to have a baby. (No other reason?) No, that's what they do it for. People who want lots of babies do it a lot, and people who wanted only one or two [babies] do it only once or twice' (English girl, 9 years).

'To have children, that's all. (No other reason?) They wouldn't want to unless they're sex mad like the Sex Pistols [a pop group]. At 25 you're starting to go off it' (English boy, 11 years).

'Having children, that's what it's all about. (No other reason?) No, that's what Father said in his sermon. God made us that way to have children' (Canadian girl, 13 years).

Not only the last girl but many others cited religious authority for their view that sex is limited to the begetting of children.

The 87% of Swedish children and the 50% of the English-speaking children who gave other reasons included sexual inter-course as enjoyment, as an expression of love, as a natural activity or as a necessity.

Sexual intercourse as enjoyment

'It makes you feel happy. It's an exciting thing and it makes your tooty [penis] feel good' (Australian boy, 13 years).

'It must be quite a thrill when you put them together. They say it gives a lot of pleasure. If that's so then people would like doing it' (English girl, 13 years).

'It kinda makes you feel good, all sort of toned up. You get rid of tensions and feel good all over afterwards' (American boy, 15 years).

'They may just like having sex. They may not want a child and they may not want to be married even. What's wrong with that?' (English boy, 15 years).

No children below the age of 9 gave opinions of this kind, and most of them responding in this way were 11 years and older, and mainly the boys. In the light of such books as *The Pleasure Bond* and *The Joy of Sex*[1] these replies are interesting. There is a clear progression with age of those who see the major reason for sexual intercourse to be enjoyment. About 75% of our Swedish 11-year-olds had this view, compared with 100% of 15-year-olds; but among Swedish 13-year-olds significantly more boys than girls offer this reason. It is perhaps understandable that fewer girls, in all countries, see pleasure as the major function, since they face more serious consequences if a pregnancy should occur. Nevertheless a sizeable and increasing proportion of teenagers of both sexes see enjoyment as the major purpose of sex apart from the procreation of children.

Sexual intercourse as an expression of love

'When you're in love you want to do it with each other. (Why?) Because it's a proof of your love. It helps you to become closer' (Australian girl, 13 years).
'There's nothing like it. It's the most binding thing there is. It means you love one another and want to be joined in one body' (English girl, 15 years).
'It's the big commitment, to give yourself to one another in the closest way you can. It's the most intimate of all human activities' (Swedish girl, 15 years).

It is very marked that in thirteen out of the sixteen age groups in all the countries sampled, a significant number of girls gave this response. The bias of boys towards sex for pleasure and of girls towards the romantic expression of love is, we believe, of considerable social significance, mirroring the differing attitudes of the sexes in adult life. Such a sharp division between the sexes is expressed clearly by a few teenagers.

'Boys like doing it more. (Why should that be so?) Oh girls have this possessive thing. They've got to feel one hundred per cent they're yours. But boys like to do it for its own sake. It's just good to do' (American boy, 15 years).
'Girls have more feeling about it. It's not just pleasure, but it's something more. It's not just giving your body. A lot of boys are just out for what they can get' (English girl, 15 years).

It is interesting that two of the most prominent popular writers about sex and the young have each provided a book which emphasise the pleasure and the responsibilities involved in the sexual act. One, called *The Facts of Love*, is about 'Living,

Loving and Growing Up' and is designed for children of 12 and older, and the other, for 15-year-olds, is called *Will I Like It?* Both are very sensible books on the question of what the ultimate sex act is for.[2] They are well worth buying for home or school libraries.

Sexual intercourse is natural

'It's instinctive. (How do you mean?) Well, all loving creatures do it. (Don't most animals do it to have young?) No, they don't know why they do it, they just have to, it's a sexual urge' (Australian boy, 13 years).
'It's the natural thing to do. (How so?) Everybody does it, well almost everyone, 'cept if you're sick or old or queer. It's men and women, based on sexual attraction' (English girl, 15 years).
'It's natural if you're married and in love. It's what makes the world go round. (How do you mean?) Well it's so, so basic. All of us have the urge and I guess you've just got to learn to handle it' (American boy, 15 years).

It is interesting that only about 4% of the respondents give this type of reply, mostly clustered around the 15-year age group. To see sex as a natural urge is quite distinct from seeing it as enjoyment or as an act of love. While it reduces sex to an animalistic instinctive act it does place it in a wider biological context; for all their observations of animal life the young obviously have not recognised it as being on the same level as human sexuality. It came through to us very clearly that most children, including the most sophisticated 15-year-olds, do not see animals and humans in a biological continuum. Some indeed express disgust because the act of sex is seen as 'behaving like animals' and so dismissed as an unworthy non-human activity which drags us down to the animal level. Such an unhealthy view can be corrected by emphasising that humans *are* animals, but enabled by higher intelligence and the development of control to lift sexuality to a higher plane. Even so, animal sexuality should not be dismissed as of a lower order, especially when one sees the devotion and the sacrifice often involved in animal mating and the rearing of their young.

Other reasons for sexual intercourse

Quite a number of the older age groups, the 13s and 15s in particular, often gave answers couched in experimental terms. People engage in sex, said some, 'to see what it's like'. Or 'It's a new experience they've never had before. They have to try it out.' Or again, 'You've got to do it sometime. They'd like to know if they are capable.'

Others said sex was an act of binding people together, not as a romantic notion or for pleasure, but more in a legal sense. 'It consolidates a marriage' says one 13-year-old, and with unconscious humour says another, 'It's a bondage in marriage'.

Three teenagers, all of them boys, gave the curious but no doubt convincing reason to them, of peer pressure being the reason for sexual intercourse. 'So they can brag about it' and 'so they can seem like everyone else' say two of them. The third is more explicit:

'It's the big thing when you're young to have sex. Some people go around wearing badges showing they're not virgins. It's a bit stupid but you feel then you've got to do it' (English boy, 15 years).

THE SEX DETERMINATION OF BABIES

Despite all the reasons for sexual intercourse given in the previous section, the vast majority of children still see the begetting of babies as its main or sole purpose. How the embryo or fetus becomes a boy or a girl is a mystery to most of the children and teenagers we questioned, and they seemed to find sex determination the most difficult of all sexual concepts to understand.

In the early years the problem is confused by many children seeing their sex identity as unstable or changing. As some of them assert, all babies are born the same sex and only later is it decided which sex they will be. One Freudian theory is that children believe all children are born boys, some having their penis removed to become girls. We did not find this belief typical of young children, the few who thought of sex instability voicing it the other way. This 5-year-old is typical.

'They are all baby girls. Then some of them are changed by medicine to boys. (What sort of medicine?) The doctor gives it to them in their milk!'

None voices any suggestion about the medicine making the penis grow, since even 5-year-olds have read adults' body and other language enough to know such talk is socially unacceptable.

Our results show that by 7 years old children have achieved the notion of sex stability or constancy, recognising that a girl is not likely to turn into a boy or vice versa. This was evident when we asked the question 'What decides whether a baby is going to be a boy or a girl?' Variants of this were 'How is it decided that a baby is going to be a boy or a girl?' and 'When a baby is started, how does it become a boy or a girl?' The question 'Who decides?' was not asked since it suggests authoritarian answers, which some children gave anyway saying it was God, Jesus, doctors or parents who were the deciders. In one case a child said it was

'the baby itself. (How do you mean?) When it's in the tummy it says, I want to be a boy or I want to be a girl. That's how it happens' (English boy, 5 years).

Because the problem posed is so difficult to answer there were a high proportion of 'Don't know', 'Can't say' and 'I haven't the faintest idea' answers, especially among the girls. Nevertheless the replies can be placed in categories which form a scale of thought, children moving up the scale with increasing age. In the first category are answers in which no causality is given at all, next are authoritarian replies, followed by descriptions of physical and psychological causes, all of which are basically non-sexual. Then there are the sexual categories which move from the behaviour of sperm and eggs, the miniaturist idea and the correct notion of interfusion or fertilisation.

Non-causal answers

'Just because' answers are typical of 5- to 7-year-olds, as the following examples illustrate:

'It's just so. It's one or the other, always has been. (How do you mean?) They've always been a boy or a girl' (American girl, 5 years).
'It's born a boy or a girl. (How is that decided?) They can tell by taking photographs' (English boy, 5 years).
'You can't tell till it comes out. (How does it become a boy or a girl?) No one knows till it comes out. Maybe it decides itself' (Australian girl, 7 years).

Plainly these children see no problem, no need to find an obvious or tangible cause. These tend to be the same children who see no point in asking 'How are babies made?' because babies have always existed.

Authoritarian answers

These tend to be given by 7- to 9-year-olds, making various authorities responsible.

'God decides what is best for the mother and father. (How does God do that?) By magic. It makes them from boy stars or girl stars' (Canadian boy, 5 years).
'The clergyman decides at the baptism, or perhaps the father decides, probably the father' (Swedish boy, 7 years).
'It's the nurse or the doctor. (How do they do it?) They inject something in the mother that decides it will have more hair and be bigger' (Australian girl, 7 years).
'Its own body, the body asks to be a boy or a girl. (How does it do that?) By telling the mother inside in some way, and she decides' (Australian boy, 9 years).
'Well there's got to be half and half in the country. (How is it decided which baby is to be a boy and which is to be a girl?) The United Nations decides them all. (How?) It's got to keep a balance. You can't have too many boys in the world' (English girl, 9 years).

So the supreme authority is the United Nations, which is brought in to control the world's sexual balance. Many of this age group are still in the manufacturers stage in explaining how babies are made, so obviously it is the manufacturers themselves who decide the sex of the new baby.

'The doctor. (How does he do it?) He asks the mother what she wants, then he tells the hospital factory to make it that way' (English boy, 7 years).

'The father buys the right seed. (How do you mean?) He orders the girl seed or the boy seed, before he puts it in the mother' (American girl, 7 years).

So the originators who make the baby have the final say by getting the right ingredients.

Non-sexual physical or psychological explanations

Some of these explanations are very simplistic, nominating the right food as the origin of sex determination; such explanations are usually given by those believing in the digestive fallacy. Obviously there is a sexist type of baby food on the market.

'It's the food mum eats. (How do you mean?) If she eats a lot of meat it'll be a boy and if she eats a lot of eggs it'll be a girl' (Australian girl, 7 years).

'It's like those minnows. If it's a girl minnow within the shell, it's a girl. If it's a boy minnow it's a boy. (How does mother get the minnows?) She eats them' (English boy, 9 years).

Maybe the last boy has got sardines and tadpoles mixed up.
   More psychological but still non-sexual are the replies which show the influence of willpower or thought control.

'Only the doctor knows. (How do you mean?) It's what you think it is. I thought it was a boy, and so did my Dad, and it was' (Australian boy, 5 years).

Or the sexes take fair shares:

'Dad decides it's going to have boys; Mum decides it's going to have girls. (How do they do that?) They take turn and turn about' (American girl, 11 years).

The peculiar behaviour of sperm or eggs

Once children know the sexual basis of conception and that this depends upon things called sperm and eggs they use these terms to explain how a baby's sex may be decided. Even if they talk of 'squirm' and 'tadpoles', many 9- to 13-year-olds develop theories based upon the peculiar behaviour of these items. One determinant suggested is the place where the sperm, cells or eggs join together or where the sperm gets into the egg.

'I don't know. (Pause) The way the cells join. They might join in different places. (How does that work?) Well, if it's on top it's a boy and if it's at the bottom it's a girl' (Australian boy, 9 years).
'It depends on the side of the egg the sperm gets in. If it's on the right it's a boy, and so on' (Canadian boy, 13 years).

Clearly some ideas of fusion are at work, but others go for speed and the angle of impact.

'It's the sperm, the one that gets there the fastest, the one with the largest tail 'cos it can swim faster. (How does this decide it's a boy or a girl?) Because when it meets the egg, it depends on which is strongest' (English boy, 13 years).
'It depends on how the squirm hits the egg. (How do you mean?) Well, if it hits it flat on and sets it off that way, it's a boy 'n if it hits it at a sharp angle it's a girl (pause), I think' (Australian girl, 11 years).
'If the egg is tough and resists it [sperm] then it's a boy; but if it lets it in then it's a girl' (English girl, 13 years).

In both these last examples there is a suggestion that weaker sperm or egg behaviour results in a girl, that is ideas of 'the weaker sex' are expressed and apparently entrenched in thinking of conception.

Miniaturist ideas

We have already seen in explaining how babies are made that those at the miniaturist stage have a simple explanation for sex determination.

'If it's a boy egg or a girl egg, a girl sperm or a boy sperm. (How does that work?) It's got a chance of two out of four what it's to be' (American boy, 15 years).

'Sperm and egg. When they meet one is dominant and becomes the baby. (How?) A dominant sperm is a boy. A dominant egg is a girl' (Australian girl, 13 years).

'I think it's the amount of hormones, if it's 51% male hormones then it's going to be a male. (How do you mean?) Like a sperm. Hormones make up the sperm' (Australian boy, 15 years).

Their ideas are on the right lines but the details become confused and incorrect in the explaining.

Chromosomal explanations

This final stage is reached by some 70% of the Swedish 13-year-olds, a stage not reached until 15 years by most of those from the English-speaking countries. Here are some replies, all of them from the 15-year-old group:

'It's DNA and that stuff. (How does it work?) When an egg with an X thing is fertilised by a sperm with a Y, the baby is male. X and X make a female' (Swedish boy, 15 years).

'There are XY boy chromosomes and XX girl chromosomes and depending on which meets which, it is a boy or a girl' (English boy, 15 years).

'Both parents decide. (How do they do that?) Through their genes. Their chromosomes mix. It's really chance, depending on the dominant chromosomes' (Australian girl, 15 years).

As in other areas, boys score significantly higher than girls in almost every age group in their insights into the sex determination question. Perhaps this reflects the bias of boys towards science, although many studies show that girls are well motivated towards biological science.

Overall, the results indicate that for both sexes the concept of genetic determination of sex at the time of fertilisation is very difficult to grasp, requiring a high level of abstract thinking in addition to formal scientific instruction.

WHY THE YOUNG NEED TO KNOW ABOUT SEXUAL INTERCOURSE AND SEX DETERMINATION

Children need to be aware of sexual intercourse as an enjoyable and fulfilling experience for both sexes, not only as a means by which babies are made. Far too many children see no further than this basic purpose, and far too many girls have a limited romantic view of sex, while boys tend to have a viewpoint limited to physical enjoyment. While the complementary nature of each sex is basic to any sexual relationship, the myth that females do not or cannot enjoy sexuality, that enjoyment is the prerogative of males, needs to be corrected. Similarly, warmth, sensitivity and the value of intimacy for men, as well as women, should be taught.

So many taboos, beginning during early childhood, surround the subject of sexual intercourse, that an open approach to the topic is greatly needed. These taboos indicate its forbidden nature, its overtones of guilt and the words used to describe it become 'dirty' words. These are most unfortunate and negative associations. Adults can help by talking about 'making love', the term causing least offence and embarrassment, as one of the most satisfying human activities, providing enormous pleasure and the result of an especially close relationship. It should also be emphasised, as most sex education courses do, that it is so important that it should be delayed until one can handle it sensitively and responsibly.

Education of the young in the genetic determination of sex is also needed, but its intrinsic difficulty probably means that its proper level is during secondary school courses. In the primary years, the important thing is to clarify the sexual nature of conception; once a more honest and accurate account of conception is given to children, they have a better foundation on which they can construct accurate ideas about sex determination.

5
HOW NOT TO HAVE BABIES

Children are not only aware of people having babies but are also conscious that some, usually married people, do not have any children or may not even want them. Television programs which children of all ages watch, from soapies to police thrillers, make frequent reference to orphans, abortions, adoptions and other means of disposing of unwanted babies. From overheard adult conversations children know the topic exists. By finding mysterious objects in bathroom or bedroom drawers some may become aware of contraception or, as one child called it, 'having contradictions'.

Publicity in newspapers and magazines does not escape the notice of children. Headlines such as 'Dead Baby Found In Dustbin', 'Abortion Clinic Raided by Police', 'Schools Fight For Contraceptive Machines' and 'Vietnamese Babies For Sale' head stories often written in sensational terms. While many children do not know the exact meaning of words such as 'abortion', 'contraception', 'birth control', 'the pill', 'adoption', 'fostering', or 'orphanages', they are words in common usage. Children are aware that they relate somehow to the outcomes of sexuality as practised by 'grown-ups'.

While surveys have been made of young people's knowledge and use of contraceptives in many countries,[1] there has been little research about how children perceive the whole area of 'not having babies' (which is not limited to ideas of preventing the making, delivery or conception of babies but includes methods of disposing of them once they are manufactured, gestated or born).

Consequently, following up questions about conception, gestation and childbirth we decided to ask the question 'What

do people do if they don't want to have a baby?' As we shall
see, most younger children interpreted the question in post-
birth terms, that is how to get rid of the baby once it is born.
We had a follow-up question about how to avoid starting a
baby, which we shall deal with later in this chapter. Meanwhile
let us see how children deal with the topic of unwanted babies.

DISPOSING OF UNWANTED BABIES

About one-third of all children who were asked about not
having babies, mainly the younger children, took the question
to mean what do grown-ups do with a baby once it's been
'ordered', or actually has been 'delivered', and the parents
change their minds. A few older children outline some of the
grim contingencies which may occur.

'Its mum and dad might be killed in a car accident the day after it's
born, so someone has to take it over' (Australian girl, 11 years).
'The mother may run off with another man to California, and the father
can't cope with small children, so he goes to the Welfare Office'
(American boy, 13 years).
'Mothers do die sometimes in childbirth. (What happens to the baby?)
Father takes it home, but if he's got other children he may not want
another' (English girl, 13 years).

All these three children talked about adoption by childless
couples, or putting them into institutions. They also faced up
to the follow-up question about how to avoid starting a baby,
designed to see what they might know about contraception.
   Not so the younger children aged from 5 to 7 years, and even
some 9-year-olds.

'The parents change their minds. They've got too many children
anyway. They give it away. (Who to?) People who want it. Them
without babies' (English girl, 5 years).
'Maybe the house isn't big enough for another baby or the father's
out of work. They sell it. It's worth a thousand dollars' (Canadian boy,
7 years).

'Sell it on the black market. (What's the black market?) That's for black babies. Some people like black babies. They look kinda cute' (American girl, 9 years old).

Others are not so imaginative and think in simpler terms of sending it back to where it comes from.

'The mother sends it back to the hospital. (What happens to the baby?) It goes back in the ambulance and waits till someone wants it' (Australian girl, 5 years).
'They ring up and say they don't want it and they take it next door and if they don't want it they send it back' (Australian boy, 5 years).
'When it's born they give it away to someone. I had a friend like that. She has brown skin and her family had white skin' (English girl, 7 years).

Or a more grisly fate awaits the unwanted baby.

'They kill it and hide it away. (How do they do that?) Don't give it any food and then put it in the dustbin' (English boy, 7 years).
'When sailors have children they drop it overboard into the sea' (Australian boy, 7 years).

By 9 years those who misinterpret the question in terms of post-natal disposal tend to think of rescuing institutions.

'They send it to an orphanage. (What is that?) It's a place you send unwanted children. There are hundreds of them there. (What kind of place is it?) Oh, they have lots of fun there, parties and they go to the circus' (English girl, 9 years).
'Is it fossicking homes? (Do you mean foster homes?) Yes fostering home. They send them there. (What sort of places are they?) Oh, they're big houses with lots of children and they all go to school together. I've seen them at my school' (Australian boy, 9 years).

Some younger children know about adoption but only vaguely, older children being more precise and informed.

'They just give it to people in the same street who haven't any babies. (Pause) It's called doption' (Canadian girl, 7 years).

'They give it an abortion. (What does that mean?) Someone wants to love the baby so they abortion it. They look after it' (English boy, 7 years).

Some confusion between the words 'adoption' and 'abortion' is quite common, as the last quotation illustrates. Others, however, are more accurate:

'They telephone the adoption agency and let them know about the baby. (What do they do?) They offer the baby to people who want one, who can't have one any other way' (Australian boy, 11 years). 'If they don't want the baby they can get it put in a children's home, or get it adopted. (What does adopted mean?) It's when parents adopt a baby and bring it up just like their own' (English girl, 13 years).

The numbers suggesting giving an unwanted baby to an institution were small, the largest being 23% of American children. Perhaps this reflects the decline in orphanages and large institutions. In children's ideas adoption outnumbers institutions five to one and is known about more accurately with increasing age. The figures overall indicate that about a third of all the children have an awareness of the full range of solutions to an unwanted baby problem (excluding contraception and abortion), however limited and confused their perception of the original cause of the problem may be.

THE SOLUTION OF ABORTION

While younger children interpret the question 'What do people do if they don't want to have a baby?' in post-natal disposal terms, most older children perceive it at both levels, i.e., as including also what to do to prevent 'starting the baby' in the first place.

But many still interpret the question in terms of terminating a pregnancy once it has started (post-conceptual as opposed to post-natal solutions). By asking later in the interview what they understood the word 'abortion' to mean and looking at their answers to the unwanted pregnancy question, we found quite considerable knowledge on the subject. At first it is confused and vague, later becoming more accurate.

Swedish children appear to be aware of post-pregnancy measures, which include abortion, earlier than their peers in other countries – 17% of Swedish 5-year-olds increasing to 43% at 7, 67% at 9 and 96-100% from 11 onwards. The comparative figures for the other countries in our study were about 9% at 5 years, 15% at 7 years, 36% at 9 years, about 60% at 11 years, about 80% at 13 and 100% at 15 years.

With increasing age the children revealed more insights and gave more accurate descriptions about induced abortions. Among those who gave more than a vague unspecified description of abortion, there were three levels of thinking.

Abortion by non-medical means

'They get rid of it. (How?) By mother doing a lot of running and a lot of jumping up and down. (What does that do?) It loosens the baby and it falls out. (Is it alive?) No, it's dead' (American boy, 9 years). 'She has an accident, like falling downstairs. You know, deliberately by mistake. (What does that do?) It shakes the baby loose from its tubes and it shrivels up and dies' (English boy, 11 years). 'My mum drinks wine every night and goes and sits in a hot bath. (What does that do?) It dissolves the baby so it comes out in her monthly periods' (Australian girl, 11 years).

Younger children get at the original artificial causes which make a baby.

'She sicks up the seed. (What does that do?) It's the seed what makes the baby, so if she's sick in the mornings she can't have one' (English girl, 7 years).

So much for morning sickness! But there are other ways of terminating a pregnancy.

'She diets. (How do you mean?) If she diets she can't get fat, so she can't have a baby' (Canadian boy, 5 years).

Dieting has another, more subtle explanation:

'She stops eating. (How does that help?) She stops the baby food. (What baby food?) The milk and eggs and stuff what makes the baby. The baby can't grow so it dies' (Australian girl, 7 years).

This is again a perfectly logical theory since if special foods make a baby, terminating the special food will get rid of the baby.

Abortion by medical but non-surgical means

These kinds of answers come mainly from 11- and 13-year-olds and mostly refer to things taken internally such as medicine, pills, tablets, or injections which somehow 'dissolve' the baby. Sometimes the pill gets confused with the contraceptive pill, as in the following:

'She takes the pill. (What does that do?) It stops her having a baby. (Can it stop the baby once it has started to grow?) That's another kind of pill. (What does it do?) It makes the baby into a kind of jelly' (English boy, 11 years).

Another version with a slightly different twist is advanced:

'It's the tablets she takes. (What kind are those?) They're conceptions tablets. (What do they do?) They make her sick and she sicks it all up. (All what?) All the baby before it's got a chance to grow. It's so tiny it comes up out of her mouth' (Australian girl, 11 years).

Yet another kind of tablet is given orally by the father.

'He gives her a tablet. It puts the baby to sleep in the mother. (How does it do that?) It's like a sleeping pill. It [the baby] probably disintegrates' (Australian girl, 13 years).

Medicine also can be given orally, usually provided or administered by a nurse or a doctor.

'The mother goes to hospital and gets some medicine stuff from the doctors. She swallows it and it kinda burns her inside stomach. (What does that do to the baby?) It burns the baby too. It's a kind of acid medicine' (American boy, 13 years).

Finally, there is the injection method, again administered by doctors.

'Yes, one can kill the baby before the twelfth week. (How is that done?) One can use a saline solution. (How?) By injection. It washes out the fetus before it grows too big' (Swedish boy, 15 years).

Abortion by surgical means

It is interesting to see that while mention is made of surgical methods of abortion by 13- and 15-year-olds, and even some Swedish children at 11, practically all describe them with negative wording, some of it in terms of faint disapproval, some of it in much stronger terms. Plainly they know in general terms what goes on and are repelled by it. They describe an operation by various means such as cutting, scraping and vacuuming:

'They operate away the fetus at a hospital, when it's very little. I think it's disgusting to throw small babies in the paperbaskets' (Swedish girl, 11 years).
'These people who say they are nurses and doctors they cut the eggs out. (How do you mean?) They operate and destroy the eggs so they die' (English boy, 13 years).
'You more or less kill the baby. You take it out of the body. (How?) The doctor puts a hook into the vagina and pulls it out. It's bound to kill the baby. It must suffer' (American girl, 15 years).
'In an abortion the baby's taken out. (How?) The doctor puts his hand into the womb and disconnects the baby. There's an injection then to cause the baby to come out' (Australian boy, 15 years).
'They have a kind of vacuum cleaner that sucks the baby out. Sounds horrible to me' (English girl, 13 years).

Although we have quoted some girls in these examples, there

are significantly fewer girls than boys who give any detailed description of abortion, particularly in the teenage years. Indeed, many of these girls' responses we had to put in 'the unspecified means of abortion' category. We expected the figures in this category to diminish with age as more specific details about abortion become known. Where the girls were concerned, however, the figures for non-specified means increased at 13 and 15 years, revealing a striking sex difference. Despite some expressed repugnance, boys had less difficulty in describing surgical abortion, whereas girls showed considerable problems in discussing it. Revulsion, moral disapproval and other negative feelings plainly inhibit girls from dwelling on the details, a reaction natural for them as the future child-bearers, in a way that is not evident for boys.

Overall, children tend to move up from non-medical types of abortion to more medicinal means and finally to see surgical methods as the major way of disposing of an unwanted pregnancy. All this however is post-conceptual activity. A more important question is how do they think of preventive approaches, namely contraception?

PREVENTIVE SOLUTIONS

Prevention answers came to the supplementary question 'What do people do if they don't want to *start* a baby?' Even if children have both post-natal and post-conceptual solutions for unwanted babies, they also may know about preventive measures, some of them invented and some based on what they have heard about contraception. We report our findings on this supplementary question as well as another question given towards the end of the interview, 'What does the word "contraception" mean?' It is important to know what teenagers know about this question, especially in view of their earlier sexual activity.

It is obvious from the answers given below that a scale from primitive to more sophisticated ideas is evident. Both in terms of their thinking powers and awareness of what is going on around them, young children are limited in their views of what can be done to avoid having babies. By arranging the scale as we have done, from 'nothing can be done' answers through to artificial means of contraception, we do not intend to show progress from bad to good methods of birth control but simply a widening awareness of knowledge from simplistic to complex methods.

Many of the answers reflect a type of fatalism that babies are meant to come and no one can do anything about it. These are the 'just because' kind of reply common to most young children.

Nothing can be done

'If God has sent a baby down it's there. (Where?) In the mother's tummy. It's just there and the baby comes' (English boy, 5 years). 'The doctor says you've got to have it. It's already been ordered' (Canadian girl, 5 years).

Medical bureaucracy obviously cannot be countermanded, as another child observes.

'The nurses will be annoyed. (Why?) They've done a lot of work on the babies. (What sort of work?) Making them in the hospital' (Australian girl, 7 years).

Nurses cannot have babies on the shelves without a suitable home to go to, any more than a supermarket can do without a reasonable turnover of goods.

This feeling of inevitability about babies is on the whole voiced by the very young, but up to 20% voice such ideas up to 9 years of age. Sweden is the exception where only 7% give such reasons at 7 years and none after that. A little different are those who see that something must be done but for them it is mainly reversing or negating the original cause, which is essentially non-sexual.

Non-sexual abstention or reversal

The children's thinking at this level is quite logical: the original cause must be removed or rendered inoperative. Some measures are religious.

'Mum tells God in prayer. (What kind of prayer?) She doesn't want a new baby just yet, so God won't send the baby down' (Australian boy, 5 years).

Some measures involve the doctors.

'The father telephones the hospital and says to the doctor, "We don't want one just yet. We're too busy with the children at Christmas!" ' (English girl, 7 years).

If the baby is seen as manufactured, the solution is simpler – don't order in the first place.

'They just wait till they're ready. (For what?) For when they want the baby to come. My mom waited for two years then told the hospital it was OK' (American boy, 7 years).

Many children who see swallowing food, eggs or seed as the beginning of babies logically see abstention from such causes as the natural way to avoid starting a baby.

'Dad waits to put the seed in. (Why?) 'Cause he doesn't want it to grow just yet. He keeps it in a pot in the shed' (Australian girl, 7 years).
'Mum is careful. (How do you mean?) About the food. She goes on a diet, no eggs, no milk, no butter and such. (Why?) They make her fat and grow the baby' (English boy, 7 years).
'They don't take the pregnant pills, that is all they do' (American girl, 7 years).

Sexual abstention

These answers range from the very simple such as 'don't get married' or the radical 'get divorced' solutions, to the more specific abstention from the sexual act. Generally these respondents see the procreation of babies as the only reason for sexual intercourse, as the following answers reveal.

'If you don't want to start one you don't get married. There's no other way. (How do you mean?) If you get married you've got to have children' (Australian boy, 9 years).
'Get divorced. (How does that do it?) Then they can't sleep together (Oh?) and make babies. That's all there is to it' (English girl, 9 years).

The older children are more specific and less inhibited about sexual abstention. Most of those who do mention it, however, reveal that it is the only effective preventive (that is, contraceptive) method they are aware of. Again, the thinking is simplistic. If this is what causes conception, then you must simply not do it.

'Don't have sex. (How do you mean?) Men and women have sex and get babies. So if you don't want one, don't do it' (Canadian girl, 11 years).
'The woman doesn't wear lipstick or scent. (What does that do?) Well, she's not so attractive then and the man won't want to do it then' (Australian boy, 13 years).
'The man doesn't put his joey in her thing. (How does that help?) So's the sperm can't swim up it and make a baby' (English boy, 13 years).

These kinds of answers decline in frequency by 11 years because children become aware of other means of contraception. About a third still give these replies at 13 years in the English-speaking groups but by this age in Sweden they have ceased. This illustrates the later report we make that the Swedish children do know about contraception much earlier than their peers in the other countries.

A few teenagers advocated abstention from intercourse and

sometimes mentioned other sexual activities such as masturbation or oral sex as a substitute.

'If you get excited then you can masturbate. (How do you mean?) That way there's no danger of the sperm getting up' (Swedish boy, 15 years). 'They can have sex with the mouth. (How do you mean?) Well, it's oral sex. They get the same feelings but don't actually have sexual intercourse' (Australian boy, 15 years).

But there were no more than a handful who voiced these ideas.

No interference with nature

Sexual abstention seems logically to give way to sexual activity which avoids conception by withdrawal (coitus interruptus), 'the safe periods' method (the rhythm method in various forms) and genital apposition. We included this last in our scale in view of evidence from an English survey that genital apposition may be a fairly widespread practice among adolescents who are sexually active.[1] One Australian 7-year-old boy, sexually very well informed, made this remarkable statement:

'The mother sleeps with her husband, but keeps her legs straight so the seed can't get in.'

Among 13-year-olds, only three boys in the five countries surveyed showed any knowledge of the three natural methods listed above, but by 15 years a few more, mainly girls, revealed that they knew about these natural methods even though the details they gave were not always correct.

'It's OK to have sex just after menstruation. (Why?) It's when the woman is less likely to be fertile' (American girl, 15 years).

This correct statement compares with another quite the opposite.

'It's safe to have sex just before menstruation. (Why?) Because there are charts showing you when it's all right' (English girl, 15 years).

In actual fact it isn't quite correct, nor is it quite so easy. The more complex basal body temperature method (bbt) is often regarded as the most reliable, but teenagers tended to talk generally of rhythm methods in very vague terms without being aware of their major variations.

Nor of course is the withdrawal method one hundred per cent safe, as these boys seem to think.

'If you pull it out in time, it's OK. (How do you mean?) Before the sperm gets out it can't get into the girl' (active Australian boy, 15 years). 'The withdrawal method. That's when you have intercourse and just before ejaculation the boy pulls the penis out. (Why?) The sperm and the egg don't meet then' (active Canadian boy, 15 years).

Surgical methods of birth control

Many children know about surgical methods of contraception, ranging from the more drastic method of castration to accurately described hysterectomy and vasectomy operations. Some know that these surgical methods can be used with males, some with females, and others, mostly 13- and 15-year-olds, know that both sexes may be candidates for surgical sterilisation. Many, however, are somewhat vague about what has to be cut.

'Oh yes, it's quite easy. The man has an operation. (What happens?) They cut him open and tie up his vocal cords' (Australian girl, 9 years). 'The mother has an operation. (What happens?) They cut her umbilical cord and tie it in a knot' (English girl, 13 years). 'It's the fallopian tubes. The surgeon does an operation and pulls them away. (Why?) So they can't produce eggs' (American boy, 15 years). 'Some men have their things cut off. (What things?) Their testicles, you know. It's mostly criminals and sex maniacs' (English boy, 15 years).

Some see a surgical operation as permanent, as in this case:

'Like when you've had six or seven kids it's time to stop' (English girl, 13 years).

Sometimes there is the innocent assumption that the operation is temporary and the tubes can easily be connected again.

'A vasectomy's only a small operation. If you change your mind it's easy to put it back the way it was' (American boy, 13 years).

Only a few Swedish children mentioned surgical methods of birth control. We assume this was because they were more familiar with the range of contraceptive devices available for both sexes, and saw no reason for the more drastic surgical methods. The few who did mention operations saw this not as a solution when the parents were young, but only after they had produced sufficient children and did not want any more.

The use of contraceptive devices

By 'devices' we include here the condom (often called a rubber, Wetcheck, Trojan or some other brand name), the diaphragm, intra-uterine devices (IUDs), the pill, vaginal spermicides (foam, cream or jelly) and pessaries. The last two, spermicides and pessaries, were rarely listed by the English-speaking teenagers, although better known to their Swedish peers.

The pill is the most widely known contraceptive device, even younger children using the term although often confused as to whether it helped prevent, produce or even abort babies. Of those who see it as a contraceptive method, few know precisely what the pill does to the ovulation of the female. Despite some detailed questioning even 15-year-olds were unaware that the pill, composed of synthetic hormones, prevents the ovaries from releasing an egg so that pregnancy cannot occur. Some had the idea it killed the egg or somehow led to early menstruation.

'The woman takes the pill. (What does it do?) It's taken once a month so the eggs can come away in the woman's period' (Australian girl, 15 years).

'She takes a pill, one every day. (What does it do?) I don't really know. Does it release the egg too soon so there's no pregnancy?' (English girl, 13 years).

However imperfectly understood, the pill is known by both boys and girls as the most widely used and most readily available contraceptive device.

Next in order of choice was the condom, known in Sweden even by some 5- and 7-year-olds. Five per cent of English girls aged 9 know of the condom but it is not known by the majority of girls in England, Australia and North America until 15 years, compared with 40% of Swedish girls aged 11 and 93% aged 13. In contrast, boys in all countries know about the condom much earlier than girls.

When questioned how the condom works, most of those who knew about it seemed to understand its function reasonably well.

'It's a kinda bag on the boy's penis, 'n when he spurts it then white goo stuff stays in the bag. It stops it going into her thing' (American boy, 13 years).

More explicit and correctly described is this:

'The condom goes on the man's penis and when he ejaculates, the semen – that's the sperm – is kept in the condom and can't get to the egg in the woman's vagina' (English boy, 15 years).

The diaphragm, also known as the Dutch Cap, is known to girls more than boys, but mainly to 15-year-olds, and how it works is grasped reasonably well. This answer is fairly typical:

'It's a kind of rubber shield wedged in the top of the vagina so that sperm can't swim up and make contact with the egg. It acts as a barrier' (Australian girl, 15 years).

Very few girls knew about IUDs (intra-uterine devices) and fewer boys, even at 15 years. None knew very precisely what the IUD device does, which is not really surprising since even the experts are unsure. All that is known is that it causes the lining of the womb to become slightly inflamed, preventing a fertilised egg from implanting itself. [2]

A good guide to how well informed teenagers are about the various contraceptive devices available is what 15-year-olds know about those devices which can be used by both sexes. There are six major types, already listed, the only male device being the condom. Most 15-year-olds knew of only two, the condom and the pill, except in Sweden where the average number of devices known was four, the condom, the pill, the diaphragm and IUDs. In Sweden about one-third of our sample knew of five devices altogether.

When totalling the results for boys and girls in each country we found the 15-year-old girls in Australia and North America the least knowledgeable and both sexes in Sweden and England the most knowledgeable. These are the two countries where sex education courses containing information about contraceptives are widely available.

WHY THE YOUNG NEED TO KNOW ABOUT 'NOT HAVING BABIES'

As part of their social education most children, even the very young, know about unwanted babies, that is babies already born who for various reasons may need to have another home found for them. A small number of children who have lost one or both parents for various reasons will be found in every classroom. In some schools where there are a number of foster homes or institutions in the neighbourhood the numbers may be quite large. Young children talk about their homes and parents a great deal both in 'news time' and during all kinds of play and work sessions.

No one is really troubled about discussing this aspect of not having babies, although it is recognised that some sensitivity is needed because of the distress it may cause to adopted, fostered and institutionalised children. Many adults however *are* worried about the other aspect of 'not having babies', and avoid telling children or even teenagers about contraception.

The Swedish practice is to include contraception in the school syllabus on 'interpersonal relations' at the most junior level, stressing the importance of not producing unwanted babies, which can be unhappy for the babies and their parents.[3] The names of the main devices are given to familiarise children with the fact that they exist. The 10- to 12-year-olds are given much more detail about contraceptives, but with the rider that at their age or even in the near future pupils should not start using them. Stress is put upon the fact that all children should be wanted when they are born, since the health of the mother and the economic well-being of the family are prime considerations. Why do the Swedes give this information from such a young age? The Swedish philosophy is simply pragmatic. Better to delay sexual intercourse, because it involves love and responsibility; but if it happens, then be responsible and informed. In the introduction to their syllabus, the Swedish authorities recognise regretfully that the age at which first intercourse occurs is getting lower, hence their deliberate inclusion of contraception as a topic from an early age, giving more information as the students increase in years.

From surveys in English-speaking countries as well as in Sweden we know that young people are increasingly active sexually at an earlier age. And many of them are not only ignorant about contraception, but about how a child is conceived, well into their teenage years. Better, we believe, to introduce the subject when the general topic of babies is being discussed and to assert the need for every baby to be born as a wanted baby, than to leave it to a time when sexual experimentation may have already begun.

Our results indicate that Australian and American teenage girls are the least aware of the implications of such early activity and the least prepared if it should happen. As few as 14% of Australian 15-year-old girls understand how to use two contraceptives, the pill and the condom, compared with about 20% of North American 15-year-old girls, the latter being among the most prone in the world to teenage pregnancy.

It was plain also that although boys knew far more about contraceptives than did girls in the English-speaking countries surveyed, the 13- and 15-year-old boys would leave it to the girl to make sure a pregnancy did not occur. Put alongside this the common teenage belief that pregnancy cannot happen at the first sexual intercourse, and we have a recipe for the high teenage pregnancy rates presently experienced in many countries. Ignorance is the major factor in causing early unwanted pregnancies.

Ignorance also of venereal diseases is an important factor to be considered. The young need to know that the pill, or any other device apart from the condom, is no safeguard against contracting disease. Publicity has been given recently in anti-AIDS campaigns about the male use of condoms as one means of safe sex, but we doubt whether this information gets to the young early enough to be effective. Given earlier maturing and earlier sexual activity in the young, this kind of information should be available to children in English-speaking countries by the time they reach the age of 10 years, and no later (see a further discussion of this in Chapter 15).

6
WEARING CLOTHES AND BEING NAKED

'If I were to walk about with no clothes on, there'd be crowds around. There'd be a riot' (English boy, 9 years).

Children as well as adults have all kinds of difficulties about nakedness. In our society the wearing of clothes is accepted for many reasons and, except in the case of very young children, to be seen without them may be a source of great embarrassment. In a recent American study 40% of young adults interviewed recalled warnings, scoldings and punishments by their parents, mother in particular, about nudity.[1] The result was that by the age of twelve 86% of boys reported being embarrassed if seen naked by a sister and 58% of girls were embarrassed when seen naked by a sister. While few boys were embarrassed at being seen naked by a brother, some 94% of girls reported embarrassment if seen naked by a brother. We found similar results for Australian families in our more recent survey.[2]

What these figures mean is that the basis of such embarrassment is sexual, stemming primarily from the prospect of the other sex seeing the sexual organs. Some embarrassment is caused to the same sex, probably because teenagers in particular are very self-conscious about their bodies and make comparisons about the size, larger or smaller, of their own sex organs. As we shall see, many adolescents, although quite normal in their growth, begin to think of themselves as physical freaks.

What is the origin of the wearing of clothes and of all these fears and embarrassments? Anthropologists advance two basic theories for the wearing of clothes. One is that clothes began to be worn in colder climates to protect the wearer from cold or in warmer climates to protect from injury or insects. The other theory, based on the idea that civilisation began in warmer climates, assumes that clothes were worn for decorative purposes, covering but emphasising the presence and size of the sex organs, thus highlighting sexual attractiveness.[3] In later civilisations and in some cultures actual nakedness was seen to be sexually provocative and so was surrounded by social taboos. Such a restraint is portrayed in the Adam and Eve myth when they are described as being ashamed of their nakedness. So shame and guilt about sexual nakedness were linked with morality and religion, a powerful authoritarian combination.

Do children in these modern times make the same inferences about nakedness? How soon in their development do they become aware of any taboos about nakedness and the necessity of wearing clothes? What reasons do they advance for what they see as the covering of their sexual parts? These and other questions we sought to answer in our interviews with the children. Consequently we asked them 'Suppose we all lived in a nice warm place or climate, should we need to wear clothes?' Whether the answer was 'Yes' or 'No' we asked the further question 'Why should that be so?'

WHY DO WE WEAR CLOTHES?

The North American and Canadian children, teenage girls in particular, appear to be the most adamant about the need to wear clothes. Among those over the age of 9, 85% saw it as an absolute necessity even in a very warm climate. Swedish children were the least concerned about wearing clothes. Even in the teenage years about half asserted it to be necessary. Thirteen-year-old Swedish girls did show some concern and so did 13-year-old English boys.

But whatever their replies, the reasons they give for their statements are of much more interest because they reveal how moralistic we have become about clothing. Using a famous American researcher's categories[4] we found there were three stages of reasoning, with most children not progressing beyond the second stage. These were first, avoidance of punishment, or self-centred pragmatism; second, conformity to social convention; third, agreement by consensus or following a universal ethical principle.

Avoidance of punishment, or self-centred pragmatism

Answers of this kind came mostly from young children who thought in terms of obedience to the adult world, punishment if they did not obey, or a self-centred concern for the practical consequences.

'Yes, because policemen might lock you up, and your father would give you a hiding. At home it's OK in the bath when you want to get clean' (English boy, 5 years).
'Mom says no, you can't do that. (Why?) You'd get the strap because it's not the right thing to do going about nakers' (Australian girl, 5 years).

These are two typical answers mentioning authority figures and possible punishment.

Concern for practical consequences can be seen in the next answers:

'No, because it'd be too hot and sweaty to wear anything. We could have our paddling pool filled' (American girl, 7 years).
'Yes, because they'd get dirty and scratched and maybe get an infection' (Swedish boy, 7 years).
'Yes, because you'd get badly sunburnt. You need to wear T-shirts. You'd go black after two or three years. (What's wrong with that?) Then you'd be mistaken for an aborigine and you couldn't get a job then. Then there are the mossies [mosquitoes]' (Australian boy, 9 years).

Some children combine avoidance of punishment with a concern for the practical consequences, as do these children giving different answers but similar reasons to justify their replies:

'Yes. (Why should that be so?) You might get sunburn and get a nasty rash. Then your mum will get you into trouble for being so careless' (English girl, 7 years).

'No. (Why should that be so?) Well, if you'd got clothes on you'd get a heat rash and then your mum would make a fuss. Better to wear no clothes and keep cool' (Canadian boy, 7 years).

It is interesting to see how mother features prominently in most of the replies. Father is mentioned only occasionally. Obviously mother is the most important arbiter in these matters as two important pieces of research in America and Britain have pointed out.[5] The researchers point out how mother appears to be the key person in the modesty training of children which includes the important tasks of toilet training and appropriate social behaviour in relation to clothing. This is especially so for girls – mothers are very firm on discipline with their daughters. In our more recent study we found 75% of mothers of children up to 12 had punished or scolded their daughters for being naked before the age of 12 and 60% of them had warned of the consequences of not wearing any clothes.

Conformity to social convention

Children have to learn what is socially acceptable, not merely how to avoid punishment or the consequences of their actions. Lawrence Kohlberg[6] writes that children are sensitive to 'Good boy: nice girl' responses, namely what pleases others; in other words, children try to live up to social expectations. At a slightly higher level is law and order thinking, involving the maintenance of social order and fixed rules for their own sake, doing one's duty and showing respect for authority. Both these reasons are given by children in late childhood and early adolescence.

'You couldn't walk up the street naked. I mean, everyone would stare at you. It's not nice. It wouldn't matter if there were only girls. If there were boys they'd be rude about it' (English girl, 9 years).

Sexual convention is very pronounced in this reply, in that the true reason for wearing clothes is to guard against the other sex.

Some children do not give clear 'Yes' or 'No' answers and the reasons they give are accordingly related to different ages or situations.

'No need to wear clothes. (Why should that be so?) It's OK if you're a baby and if it were hot. But if it were hot and you had to go to school, you'd need to wear clothes. (Why?) The others would laugh. It's just normal to wear clothes. Everyone does' (American girl, 11 years).

Although to be laughed at or ridiculed is a kind of punishment it is a consequent reaction of peers, not of authority, and in her answer she reflects more a concern for social conformity in following what 'everyone does'. The law and order argument is given by another child:

'There's laws against it. (Against what?) Going around with no clothes on. It'd cause traffic jams and accidents I mean, if you saw a naked girl walking along the street. If everybody did it we couldn't keep order' (English boy, 11 years).

Again the appeal is to law and order, both words actually being used. But in these days when nudity is allowed in certain places, even this has to be limited:

'Yes. It's rude. You can only go to certain beaches so they can get tanned all over. They're showing all their personal things. It's got to be kept under control' (Australian boy, 15 years).

Even in enlightened Sweden there are limits:

'Yes, you can't simply be naked. That is not educated' (Swedish boy, 13 years).
'Yes, because we wouldn't dare to show our genitals to each other' (Swedish girl, 13 years).

All these reasons reflect an inflexible adherence to rules, a conventional acceptance of what is rather than what should be. The vast majority of children in middle and late childhood and also in their adolescence respond in this way.

Agreement by consensus or following a universal ethical principle

At this third stage even adolescents have difficulties. It takes quite a high level of reasoning, and intelligence, to see that the wearing or not of clothes can be decided by consensus. One must be aware of a relativism in personal values and also between cultures to see that laws may be changed on rational consideration. People are not free to do what they like but agreement in the form of consensus can allow greater freedom to individuals. At a higher level still there are the dictates of conscience based upon ideas of the equality of individuals and the application of universal principles. Not surprisingly, among 15-year-olds only 28% of the English children reached this stage of post-conventional thinking, 42% of the North American children and 50% of the Swedish children. What is surprising is that 80% of the Australians did reach this stage, perhaps because of the outdoor life of most Australians and the growing practice, based upon consensus, of acceptable nudity at many beach resorts.

We quote below not only 15-year-olds but other ages who give these types of replies:

'No, because everyone's the same. If it was hot you wouldn't need to wear clothes, because everyone's the same. (Men and women?) It wouldn't matter if everyone agreed to it' (Australian girl, 9 years).
'Say we had another Ice Age we'd all wear clothes for sure. But if the opposite happened and we had a Heat Age everyone would agree clothes weren't necessary. It's all a matter of people agreeing' (Canadian boy, 11 years).

These are clearly consensus answers, whereas what follows are more the appeal to conscience based upon a wider principle.

'I don't think you should be ashamed of your bodies. They are all the same. Adam and Eve didn't wear clothes. (But didn't they feel ashamed?) Oh, that's an old-fashioned story' (American girl, 13 years).
'Some believe you shouldn't wear clothes, like nudists, and some believe you should. People should be free to choose' (American boy, 13 years).
'Everyone's the same and it's no use hiding it. The only reason for clothes is for warmth, so they can be discarded if they are warm. It depends on what sort of person you are. If you don't want to show your body off, it's up to you' (Australian girl, 15 years).
'Most moral laws would inhibit it. The concept of shame has been put in people's minds, and this has restricted them' (English boy, 15 years).

And a judicious statement is made by a 15-year-old English girl:

'It's not shameful to be naked, but it's usually wise to wear clothes.'

Why is it that so many teenagers have difficulty reaching the third stage? Well, research has shown that many adults have difficulty too. This is true especially where the question becomes a moral one. Most people play safe and go for a conventional answer based on 'everybody does it' thinking. It is also complicated by the fact that thinking in terms of consensus or principle requires abstract thinking whereas most people are more confident thinking in concrete terms. Adolescents are no exception to this.

Because the question about wearing clothes did not ask directly why the exposure of the sex organs in particular should be forbidden, we asked a further question: 'Some people feel shy or funny about certain parts of the body. Why should this be so?' We did not need to define what we meant by 'certain parts of the body' since children knew what was meant immediately. Young children, we found in trial interviews, did not understand the word 'embarrassment' so we used 'feeling shy' or 'funny' which they well understood. Their responses to this question are very interesting.

THE NEED TO COVER THE SEX ORGANS

So far in discussing the wearing of clothes, some children had mentioned, although only indirectly and usually not calling them by name, the sexual parts of the body. Most had not. But following immediately after the discussion on the wearing of clothes, children found the right context in which to talk more freely. Even so they still frequently observed the social taboos of not naming the sexual organs.

We found the same three stages of thinking about this problem as with the wearing of clothes. The moral considerations were even stronger.

Letting anyone see your sexual parts is punishable

Even as young as 5 the children have been conditioned to think in these negative terms.

'People shouldn't show them. (Why not?) Because they're shy. (Pause) You'd get smacked by Mum and when Dad gets home he'd smack you too' (Australian girl, 5 years).
'Because windows might be showing and some people might see you and Mummy might smack you' (American boy, 7 years).

The implication of these answers is that within the family it may be all right, but with those outside it is not, an idea which is quite realistic, as this explicit example shows:

'We're not shy when it's bathtime. My brother and sister and me all have a nice bath together. But if we've got visitors we've to get into 'jamas before we see them. (Why?) 'Cause they're not supposed to see our thingos' (English girl, 7 years).

But this is limited to younger children. Older children soon begin to feel that it's all right when you are young but not if you have a sibling of the other sex.

'In the family it may be OK when you're all young kids. But when

96

you get older you don't all bath together any more. (Why not?) As a boy I don't want my sister looking at me seeing what I've got. (Why not?) My folks would punish me, think it's rude' (Canadian boy, 9 years).

Here is how an 11-year-old girl reports how she feels on these matters.

'When we were small my brother and me played around with nothing on. Now we're older we've got to be more careful. (How do you mean?) We get dressed separately. My brother's got very shy and won't let me in the bathroom. Dad's told us to.'

Perhaps it is partly natural reticence but plainly much of it is imposed by parents on growing children without explanation. Children naturally infer what the taboos are and carry them through into their adolescence.

Some children swing between the fear of being punished and more pragmatic considerations:

'They don't want to be seen. They'd maybe get into trouble with their mum and dad. Anyway they might get hurt. (How do you mean?) They might get sunburn or get bitten by a snake there. (Where?) On your thingummy-jigs' (English girl, 9 years).

It's normal to be embarrassed

Most children accept that it is normal to be embarrassed at nudity, because it means other people, including their own family, seeing the sex organs. Again, while natural reticence may be desirable some of the reasons used are unfortunate.

'They don't want to show them off. (What?) Those parts that are smelly and ugly. And you'd be showing off, you'd wear something over them. (Why?) They'd not like to show their dinkle' (English boy, 7 years). 'Because others would laugh at them. It's not funny to me. Why, my mom takes her clothes off and I'm taking a nap, and I peep and I don't laugh' (American boy, 7 years).

The taboos are repeated as at the earlier stage that it is the other sex one has to worry about, not one's own.

'Men and women are different and it's normal to be careful and feel shy. If it's just women together it's all right' (English girl, 9 years). 'When boys are in the shower at school after football that's OK. (Why?) Well they've all got the same things, penis things, and no one notices' (Australian boy, 9 years).

But soon even with one's own sex the embarrassments begin to occur. With the onset of pubertal growth children begin to make comparisons, even if 'they've all got the same thing'.

'Maybe they don't like their own body, they think they look awful. They have lots of freckles on them, and maybe their bust is too small or too large' (English girl, 11 years).
'When you're changing for gym the other blokes make remarks about your balls and stuff. If you are big it's very uncomfortable when they start joking' (Australian boy, 13 years).
'No, I'm not beautiful and I feel safer with my clothes on. You may have too big breasts and be an early maturer, and you don't want to be teased' (Swedish girl, 15 years).

Many of these answers show the growing self-consciousness of teenagers as their bodies change. Is this self-consciousness natural? It probably is, but it is also probably encouraged by the fact that teenagers generally do not know what normal development is. Both small and large penises and breasts are within the range we call normality, and ignorance of this leads to the feeling among most adolescents that they are physical freaks.

Others come back to a more conventional reply, often citing the reasons of law and order in a different form.

'It's in the interests of privacy. You don't show your sex organs. (Why not?) We like to reserve certain things to ourselves. They tried topless dresses and they didn't take on because people don't like it' (Australian girl, 13 years).
'Everyone wears clothes now and they think it's rude to show the

privates. They probably made a rule a long time ago which spread. (Why?) Don't know the original reason but you've got to accept it' (English boy, 11 years).

A healthy view of the problem

More open and less embarrassed feelings are expressed by some older children and adolescents who see embarrassment as often irrational and imposed by a society which has an unhealthy view of sexuality. Or some see a more rational basis than social convention for sex taboos about revealing the sex organs. This third stage of reasons is reached by about a third of the 15-year-olds in Australia and Sweden, and by only about a quarter of the 15-year-olds in England and America. Here are some examples from a range of ages.

'After several generations people wouldn't be embarrassed, like the Africans, they're not. (Don't some Africans cover up certain parts of the body?) Yes, but they live in places where whites have taught them to be ashamed' (English boy, 11 years).
'You were born with nothing on. There's no reason to be embarrassed. But if people haven't gone naked for a long time, since civilization [began], it could be regarded as wrong' (Australian boy, 11 years).

The argument that people have been indoctrinated into embarrassment is often made. This 15-year-old is typical:

'They're ashamed because they're taught it's rude to show the parts of a man or woman. They're told they are *private* parts. And many people don't understand their sex organs and won't show them' (American girl, 15 years).

The argument that people may be truly embarrassed for rational reasons is advanced clearly by this 15-year-old:

'Boys might have an erection or girls might have a period. It would be embarrassing. Normally we don't go to a formal dance with nothing on. But it's been going on so long, wearing clothes, because Europeans started in a cold place' (Australian boy, 15 years).

'When you're in close contact with the opposite sex you feel stimulated. (How do you mean?) Your penis stands up and you wouldn't want them to see that. I'm told girls' nipples do the same. That's why they're covered up, it could be real embarrassing' (American boy, 15 years).

Both kinds of explanation, the growth of tradition which may be broken, and the real basis for sexual embarrassment, go beyond the conventional views expressed at the second stage. Again the level of thinking required is extremely demanding and it is not surprising that so few achieve this third stage.

WHY CHILDREN NEED TO THINK ABOUT CLOTHING AND NAKEDNESS

We would like to make it clear at this point that we are not propagandists for universal nudism. We do recognise that nudist colonies have the right to exist, provided they are in areas where they do not cause offence to others. Similarly nudist beaches, now on the increase in Australia, are a healthy development for those who wish to use them. The wearing of clothing clearly has its conventions, which change according to fashion. The time when a lady's ankle had to be covered has long been overtaken by the mini-skirt and other more revealing developments. But for most people social and sexual conventions have to be observed and parents, especially mothers, still have the difficult task of 'modesty training' for their children.

The problem is that children are often inducted into the conventions in a negative manner involving warnings, scoldings and punishments, which encourage them to see nakedness as some kind of shameful condition. Associated with this negativism is the view of the sexual organs as dirty, ugly, embarrassingly private and on all occasions something to be guilty about.

What are the needs of our children, where clothing and nakedness are concerned? They are

- a healthy openness to nakedness within the family in the early years, especially at bathtime, during the summer and at the beach;
- a need to see the sex organs as normal functional parts of the body of which we need not be ashamed;
- a gentle induction, free from repressive associations, about the need to respect others' feelings, explaining why older people, relatives or visitors may be concerned at seeing nakedness;
- some sensitivity in the pubertal years to the self-consciousness felt about the growing sex organs, with some information about the wide range of what is normal;
- within the family, an acceptance of the need for privacy, especially when and if requested by siblings of the other sex.

Overall, if these needs can be met children will grow through childhood and adolescence and into young adulthood with a more wholesome view of the human body.

One important problem related to all we have discussed on this topic is warning children about sexual abuse by adults. As we report in Chapter 11, most adults who sexually abuse children are known to them, and may even be a member of the child's own family. How can we help children understand what may happen to them and help them to protect themselves? As we have pointed out in discussing Protective Child Sexual Abuse Programs, the first basic instruction is to teach children that they have a right to say 'No' to anyone who wishes to touch them. In this sense we teach children that the sex organs in particular are private parts and children have the right to refuse anyone who wishes to see, touch or manipulate them.

There is no inherent contradiction between teaching a child to say 'No' in such circumstances and the needs of children to see their bodies in a wholesome light and to assert their rights to privacy. We shall discuss these and related matters when we come to look in more detail at children's experiences of sexual abuse in Chapters 11 and 12.

7
WHAT THE YOUNG WANT TO KNOW
ABOUT SEX

'I'm not ignorant. I just don't know' (English boy, 11 years).

The list of sexual matters of which children are ignorant, or at best only partially informed, is a very long one. Previous chapters have outlined some of the ways in which this ignorance distorts what should be a happy and wholesome view of sexuality for the growing child.

Despite their ignorance, all the children we talked with were making honest attempts to get at the truth about many aspects of sex. We have seen how they invent mythologies to explain how babies are made and how they are born, and their partial interpretations about many other sexual matters. It is not only philosophers and deep thinkers who pursue a relentless quest for the truth. Children too are concerned to know and often express their anger and disgust that they are so often and so seriously deceived about sex by adults.

'My parents were so nervous about it all, it is unbelievable. I mean, I'd ask a simple question about my penis – I think I was about 4 years old – and they'd go red in the face and mumble and avoid the subject. I soon learned they'd tell me nothing or maybe didn't know themselves' (Australian boy, 13 years).

'The first sex education we had at school was when I was 13. And I began my periods when I was 11. My mum had told me a little about the bleeding but it was such a shock. It happened during the night and I felt so ashamed. There ought to be a law saying children must be told' (English girl, 15 years).

In some countries or states some laws do exist making it

obligatory to provide sex education for children, but in many places it is left too late, in the secondary school stage, or it is not provided at all because nerveless politicians have bowed to noisy narrow-minded bigots. Often the politicians take a middle road, allowing each individual school to decide, so each school in turn may become a battleground instead of operating under a centrally decided law which makes it the right of every child to know. Children are only dimly aware of these battles but one thing is certain. They themselves, the clients or consumers, really do want to be rescued from their ignorance.

'It really is laughable in this day and age how the grown-ups are so secretive. Everyone has to know about sex sooner or later if the world is to go on. When I'm a parent I'll tell them from an early age. (When?) As soon as they start to ask questions' (Canadian girl, 11 years).

Kids have some very interesting ideas about sex education, when it should begin and who should give it. But first let us see what it is they want to know.

WHAT THEY WANT TO KNOW

Towards the end of the interview we asked the children 'What is the most important thing a boy (girl) needs to know about sex?' For some younger children the question did not make much sense, even though we changed the phrasing to knowing about babies, or other matters they had discussed.

Many 5-year-olds gave answers such as 'What's bad for your teeth', 'How to hold a baby and not drop it', and 'How not to fall down and hurt my knee'. Some were a little nearer the mark but still not on the sexual target when they said 'How to get married', 'What to eat if you want to have a baby' or 'How to help your wife'.

Most children from 7 years on had some notion about what the question meant. The older the children the more precise they were about what they should know about sex. Many of the teenagers did know many sexual facts by this time but regretted they had not been told earlier, saving them much bewilderment and needless worry.

'We had the first real sex course last month given by a doctor. It told us all about the human body, girls and boys. I already knew most of the facts. It came about five years too late' (American girl, 15 years).

What were the most important things about sex these children felt they should know?

Body changes at puberty

Teenagers in particular voiced a concern to know how their developing bodies would grow and change. To be prepared for such changes was an idea implicit in what they said:

'It's just daft to be ignorant of what's happening to your body. You're no longer a child, but you're treated like one. No one tells you about your sex organs and the sort of feelings you get' (English boy, 15 years).
'I got really worried when hair started to grow under my arms and between my legs. I guess I was an early developer 'cause I worried about it when I was around 10. My mom laughed and just said, "Now you're growing up". But I didn't know what she meant' (American girl, 13 years).

Few parents and fewer teachers seem to think it important that pubertal children become informed about what is happening to their bodies. Many teenagers had heard the terms slow and early developers, often accidentally from adult conversations:

'My mum said to my aunty one day, when I was in the next room and the door was open, I was a slow developer. I got real worried, thought it was my brain or something and I was going to be a right moron' (very bright Australian girl, 13 years).
'I was told at school by a well-meaning teacher that I was an early developer. She said I could have babies sooner and I got into a panic thinking I was going to have one soon. I was about ten at the time' (English girl, 15 years).

These youngsters could have had fewer anxieties if instead of casual comment some effort had been made to show them the range of normal development and what growing into adolescence really means.

Sex differences

Pre-teenage children had other concerns, not least to be told what the real differences were in men and women, namely sex differences.

'I knew for a long time about how the bodies of girls and boys weren't the same. But we ought to know all about it much earlier. (When?) Oh, when you're a small child. I'd like to know the real names now' (Australian boy, 9 years).

Presumably this boy means the real names for the sex organs, which a chance remark revealed he regarded as dirty. A more forthright and informed girl who knew the correct terms still wanted more details.

'It's silly all this secrecy. A man's penis and a girl's vagina need special care. I'm told if you don't keep them clean you can get disease. We need telling all about that' (American girl, 11 years).

This next teenager looking back at his childhood years was astonished how long sex differences had been kept from him.

'Differences between men and women. It's amazing how long I was in total ignorance about that. For a long time I thought it was how people dressed, then I realised it was what was there between the legs that was different. I once asked my parents and there was a terrible silence' (English boy, 15 years).

Menstruation

A few boys said they would like to know about this feature of female growth, but not one boy except in Sweden rated it as the most important. Not surprisingly, the vast majority of girls rated this as number one or very high on their list. The most graphic comments come from the teenage girls who had gone through the experience, although a few younger ones – the rare exceptions – voiced their need before it happened. These mainly are the girls already prepared and informed by their mothers.

'Your period. You need to know what to expect. My mother told me I can expect it any time now and I carry around a sanitary towel just in case. I'm a bit nervous about it though' (Australian girl, 11 years).

She might be nervous, but hers is nothing like the plight of some older teenagers looking back on their worrying experience of the first menstruation.

'Periods. My mother was stupid, kept saying I'll tell you when you're a bit older. I knew something was going to happen but didn't know what. Then right in the middle of gym (at school) I started to bleed. I thought I'd torn something inside and I lay in the sick room worried to death, until a teacher came and told me what to do' (Canadian girl, 15 years).

So many mothers are embarrassed about discussing menstruation and are also unaware of the earlier maturing of most adolescent girls, that they do delay. We would like to report that these were rare cases, but unfortunately they were all too common. This 13-year-old girl is fairly typical:

'When you menstruate. Mine was bloody [sic] awful. I didn't know what to expect, then suddenly when I was out shopping with a friend, it happened. I thought I'd need an ambulance, but the lady in the dress shop went to the chemist's [pharmacy] next door and fixed me up. I was shaken and frightened' (Australian girl, 13 years).

This girl's mother, so the girl reported, had not told her about menstruation because her daughter 'might get worried about it' – nothing to the anxiety experienced at the time and the shame of being informed by an unknown lady in a dress shop.

When boys did put menstruation on their list of things

106

important to know it was usually in terms of curiosity or wanting to know 'how the other half lives'. Swedish 13- and 15-year-old boys were the only male group of any size who wanted to know. Significantly boys did not list at all their own equivalent to the girls' menstruation, the appearance of nocturnal emissions, often called 'wet dreams' (more of this omission later).

Breast development

Many girls voiced concern that they had known little about the growth of their breasts as this change was happening. They report it as a source of some anxiety not only because their growth was sometimes unexpected or unexplained but also because of the accompanying greater sensitivity experienced.

'Breasts; what they are and what they're for. Mine grew very quickly from the time I was about 9 or 10. They sort of tickled a lot and sometimes it was uncomfortable. Mum sort of said it was to do with babies and such, but it was confused and I was embarrassed for a long time' (English girl, 15 years).

'Bosoms. Suddenly I grew these bosoms and I didn't know why. A friend of my mother's one day talked to me about growing up. She was very kind and calmed me down when I said all the boys were looking at me. She said, "That's OK, it's the way women attract men. You've to be grateful to have good boobs" ' (American girl, 15 years).

Many girls expressed fears, not about the actual development of breasts, but about being normal. They were concerned that they would have breasts too small or too large. So many were worried about being seen as freaks and most had only vague ideas about what should be considered 'normal' in breast development.

Conception

The importance of knowing about conception was voiced at all ages, but only rarely was the word 'conception' itself known or used. Children who had a non-sexual explanation for how babies are made would talk in non-sexual terms.

'How you get the seeds. (What seeds?) To get the baby growing. You can't have the baby without them so you've got to know the right shop' (Canadian boy, 5 years).
'About the eggs. (What about the eggs?) Well, what to do with them. Mother's got to eat them an' have a baby. They've to get the right ones' (English girl, 5 years).

Information about what to purchase and where to buy it is not the only concern. What to do with the seed, the eggs, the baby-making foods once you have them is seen as important.

'How Dad's got the seed in Mum. (How do you mean?) How he gets it in her. To tell him to get her to swallow it at night' (Australian boy, 7 years).
'Mum and Dad need to know what food to eat. (What food?) For making babies out of. If they don't know they can't have a baby, can they?) (English boy, 7 years).

It seems that these younger children are more concerned that their parents receive instruction than the children themselves. Older children who have grasped that something sexual must occur for conception to take place see it as something they as children should know about.

'What happens when they join belly-buttons. (How do you mean?) How the father's seed gets through into mum's tummy. How the white stuff comes' (American girl, 9 years).

Others among the reporters are curious about sperm and eggs, and want to know in more detail what happens to make conception possible.

'I'd like to know what happens to make a baby. OK, I know the man's sperm gets in her stomach and grows into a baby. What happens to the sperm? It turns into an egg doesn't it?' (American girl, 11 years). 'I think we should be told about conception, how it happens. I'd have liked to have known about it a lot earlier. It's not dirty, it's really quite beautiful to know how life begins. It's kept secret far too long' (Australian boy, 13 years).

Sexual intercourse

Boys in particular express the need to know 'how to do it' although some girls also feel it to be important. One boy puts it crudely but succinctly:

'How to do it. (What do you mean?) How to fuck. Why everyone's so secretive I don't know. You've got to do it, or the world would die out' (English boy, 15 years).

Or more polite, but still revealing a genuine natural interest, is the answer

'What men and women do together. (What is that?) How to make love. (Pause) People won't talk about it except in dirty jokes. It's very difficult to know exactly what to do' (Australian boy, 15 years).

As it happens, the last boy quoted knew all there was to know. But he said he had to find out from many different sources, the principal one being an encyclopedia.

Australian and English boys were significantly more numerous than the girls in listing sexual intercourse as a major topic to know about. Swedish teenage boys also showed strong interest.

Contraception

Not until we reached the 15-year-olds were there significant numbers listing the topic as important. At 13 years there were few showing an interest and at 15 girls in Australia (25%), boys in England (35%) and boys in America (25%) were by far the more curious. Compared with this, Swedish 15-year-olds showed much more concern, 47% each for boys and girls, perhaps reflecting the fact that both sexes have been taught about contraception for many years and see it as a shared responsibility, not the responsibility of one sex only.

'Birth control. It's an important subject, 'specially if you don't want to get a girl pregnant' (active American boy, 15 years).
'You've got to know about contraceptive things. Otherwise you might land in a whole heap of trouble. If a girl doesn't do something, like take the pill, the boy may not do anything, thinking the girl does' (active Australian girl, 15 years).
'They ought to make condoms free, or in machines. It's very embarrassing going into the chemist's [pharmacy], there might be a girl serving at the counter' (English boy, 15 years).

Those who are not sexually active at the age of 15 still stress the need to know about contraception. Girls especially are well aware of the dangers of teenage pregnancy. But still the figures are disappointingly low in the light of the lowering age for first intercourse.

Pregnancy, gestation and birth

Few children listed these topics as important for them to know about. For most, having babies is in the realm of grown-up life, the concern of parents, reflecting an assumption that there is time enough to learn about such matters. Time enough for most, but for some 10 per cent in their teenage years these will become important matters sooner than they think.

SEXUAL TOPICS NOT LISTED AS IMPORTANT TO KNOW ABOUT

There were several topics not listed or mentioned by only a few as important topics they felt they need to be taught. Among the topics missing were masturbation, wet dreams, sexually transmitted diseases, courtship behaviour and parenting.

Masturbation

This is a topic most young people are worried about, evoking feelings of guilt and shame, particularly among boys. Yet this was not listed because, we believe, it is a taboo subject with a long history of social sanctions. When adults talk about masturbation to adolescents as 'self-pleasuring', that is, as a legitimate substitute for the sexual act and an alleviation of sexual tensions, there is considerable relief expressed in knowing that it is a widespread 'normal' activity.

Wet dreams

These occurrences, also called night or nocturnal emissions, are the involuntary release of semen mainly during sleep, which signal the maturing of the male. These are universal happenings, few boys not experiencing them. We know from informal discussion with many hundreds of boys that like masturbation they cause feelings of guilt. Because they leave stains on the bedsheets they are condemned by some parents as 'dirty' activities. The need for boys to be prepared beforehand for this occurrence is self-evident, but not one male interviewed voiced the need.

Probably so many negative feelings are invoked, as with the topic of masturbation, that there is a reluctance to raise the subject. For some boys we know the shock of first wet dreams and the feelings of shame that follow are similar to the reactions of girls unprepared for their first period.

Sexually transmitted diseases

There was a total silence on this increasingly important sexual topic. While cases of syphilis among teenagers have not increased in recent years, gonorrhoea has shown considerable increases.[1] There are also alarming increases in herpes and, of course, the disturbing increase in AIDS (Acquired Immune Deficiency Syndrome). The first has consequences which last for years and the second results in many cases in premature death. Reliable statistics on teenage herpes and AIDS are not yet available but with increased earlier sexual activity and still a widespread ignorance regarding appropriate protection, teenagers are seen as particularly prone to sexually transmitted diseases. Yet no boy or girl in our survey listed any disease or venereal diseases generally as important.

Courtship and premarital behaviour

A few teenagers at 11 and 13, particularly among the Americans, list courtship practices as important, perhaps because dating occurs earlier there. But what to do when going out with the other sex, the courtesies to be observed, the dos and don'ts, are generally not regarded as vital. Premarital sexual behaviour is a total blank, and that includes not just early dating but regular dating with the same person. Young people seem to be in great need of some guidance in this area, but there is no indication that they feel themselves to be in need of it.

Parenting

Perhaps caring for babies and helping children to grow up seems very remote from the lives of teenagers. Yet some 10% of girls will be faced with the prospect of becoming parents before they reach the age of 20. No teenager voiced concern about knowing the skills and duties of parenting, although there are some school courses developing this topic especially in home economics for girls.

Overall it is evident that children and teenagers do want to know about sex; their major concerns are how the body works, sex differences, menstruation, breast development, conception and sexual intercourse. These are wise observations about what they need to know, although other important topics such as contraception and pregnancy, gestation and birth are comparatively low on their list of what is important. What they omit from their list is disturbing. These include masturbation, wet dreams, sexually transmitted diseases, and courtship and parenting, all topics relevant especially in the teenage years.

Two matters stand out from the children's remarks about the topics they list as important. First, if they have received any formal sex education at school, most of the topics they believe to be important have not been dealt with at all or only dealt with late in their teens, when the urgent reasons for teaching most of them had passed. Second, and because of this experience, children do want sex education provided and they want it much earlier than a nervous adult community thinks appropriate. Let us now see exactly what children think about sex education, by whom and when it should be provided.

CHILDREN'S SOURCES OF SEX INFORMATION

It is clear that children believe that they should ideally be told about sex by their parents. But they quite forthrightly speak of their parents as limited or unwilling or both, and so the children generally hesitate to ask questions and parents in turn hesitate to tell their children.

'I wouldn't ask them 'cos it's supposed to be a secret. They won't tell anyone' (Australian girl, 5 years).
'I'd rather not tell them. It'd be rude' (English boy, 7 years).
'They wouldn't tell you. You're too young to know this. You'd get a smack' (Australian boy, 9 years).
'My mum won't tell me. She says I'm too young and she won't tell me until I'm 13' (English girl, 9 years).
'My dad hasn't got time. He's always listening to the radio and we're not allowed to talk' (Canadian boy, 11 years).
'No, not my parents. They'd probably ask me why. Dad would probably go against it till I'm older' (Australian boy, 13 years).
'Not usually. We don't talk about it in the family. It would have

to be very serious' (American girl, 13 years).
'They'd not really listen even if we did ask, and we'd all be embarrassed' (English boy, 15 years).
'No. I've got to live with them. What will they think of me if I ask all these questions?' (American boy, 15 years).

Yet this last American boy said he could talk about sex and get information from his girlfriend's mother.

Dad is the great ogre, apparently, in this area, not very forthcoming about sex and prone to become negative if any questions are asked. About 3% of children rated their fathers comfortable about discussing sex with them, although in Sweden the percentage was higher (9%). Even then, fathers may take their sex education rather casually:

'Dad tells me. He gives me his old copies of *Playboy* magazine for me to see' (American boy, 11 years).

Although *Playboy* contains only a mild form of titillation it is disturbing to think of an 11-year-old boy using such a source for sex education.

Girls, especially in their teenage years, use mothers as their major source of sex information, between 22% and 32% of them doing so. But a much higher percentage use Mother as a confidant and say they feel comfortable asking her questions about sex.

'My mum would know. She's had babies and gone through having periods. She's more reasonable than Dad and takes it seriously' (English girl, 11 years).
'Mum's more understanding. She listens. I'd be a bit jumpy but I think she'd understand. Dad would just think I'd been mucking around' (Australian boy, 13 years).

Nevertheless, children are aware that the questions to be asked are limited by Mother's knowledge and education and her willingness to talk about what is often a touchy subject.

Boys are in a particularly difficult situation. In discussing whom could they ask questions about sex, far fewer boys said they felt free to ask their mothers, especially as they get older. Less than half the boys can ask their mothers and less than a quarter their fathers. Whom can they ask?

It is interesting that parents rate only moderately as sources of sex education, some 19% of our sample mentioning them performing that function. But teachers are much more significant, at 32%. Swedish teachers, working in a system which has compulsory sex education, rated especially high in this respect; England, where sex education is reasonably widely available in school, shows teachers mentioned by 28%, and Australia and America, where sex education is very patchy, show teachers at 19%.

Among other sources from which children claim to get their sex information are the media – TV, films, books, encyclopedias and magazines – representing about 20% of their major sources. Friends rank low at about only 8%, most children recognising that they only share misinformation and gossip rather than accurate information. One cautionary feature about discussing sex with friends, many children said, was

'You've got to pretend you know. Because if you show you don't know, it gets around the school. Even if you don't know, you pretend you do' (American girl, 11 years).

CHILDREN WANT SEX EDUCATION AT SCHOOL

Because children generally perceive their sources of sex information as inadequate, we asked them if children should be taught about sex and when and where. Almost 100% of the children said they wished to be taught, the negative ones tending to be the 5- and 7-year-olds who did not understand the question. Many of these, and even a few older children, voiced some of the adult misgivings about sex education.

'The mother may not want the child to know' (English boy, 7 years). 'If you look at pictures, you might kiss it' (English boy, 7 years). 'No. Because if they do they'd tell others. Boys think it dirty' (Swedish girl, 7 years).

'No. My mother wouldn't let me know about babies and I've never yet found out' (American boy, 9 years).

When the children were asked if sex education should be taught in school, the answers were still overwhelmingly supportive. Negative ideas are disappearing by 9 years, when about 70% approve, about 90% support the idea by 11 years (the lowest figure is 70% for Australian 11-year-olds), and moving to 100% in all countries at 13 years and older.

'When should such lessons begin?' we asked the children. The results are interesting, especially the comments from Swedish children. The following perceptive comments were made by Swedish teenagers:

'At 4 in kindergarten, when they start wondering. It's important not to lie about anything.'
'They are all ready at 2 when they ask "what has father got there?".'
'Seven years old when you can understand it.'
'Yes. Nine years, not sooner, you must know a little first.'
'Yes at 10, otherwise you'd know nothing when you menstruate.'
'You should start at 5 years old. Then give them the facts at about 10 years.'
'At 10 in school, but mother and father must certainly tell about it earlier at about 7 or 8 years.'
'At 5 to 6 years. It varies with the child's maturity.'

These opinions are from children who have received sex education from 7 years old, most of them even earlier in kindergarten and in the home, and whose parents are more confident and less inhibited about the subject because they themselves have had such courses in their childhood.

Although less articulate than their Swedish peers, the English-speaking children have similar opinions. They overwhelmingly want sex education to start in the primary or elementary schools. The only hesitation is among North American 15-year-olds, whose experience of sex education courses, if any at all, has been restricted to the later part of their secondary schooling. These vote safely for the start of sex education to be in secondary schools, following their own experience. American

116

children too show themselves to be more aware of parental opposition to sex education in the public school system.

The children's judgment that sex education of some kind should start in the primary school is consistent with the research findings about earlier sexual maturing we outlined earlier in this book's Introduction. In this they seem to be wiser than their elders, who have tended to think that the secondary or high school is the appropriate level.

WHY PRIMARY SCHOOL CHILDREN SHOULD KNOW ABOUT SEX

For most children the primary school years are a settled period of growth until pubertal changes begin for some as soon as 8 years, for others by 9 or 10. Most experts indicate that it is in these settled years that children want to learn about sex and are capable of receiving information on this subject, as they are avid and enthusiastic collectors of information in most other subjects. We have seen that they have already acquired a great deal of sexual knowledge but much of it partial or misinformed. They have to complete the picture of sex differences, sex relations, conception, pregnancy and other vital matters from their imagination or by sharing ignorance with their friends. Their innovative sexual ideas may be amusing but they do interfere with a more intelligent understanding of sexuality in later years. In many cases they are serious impediments to learning.

Children are fortunate indeed if they have parents who have wisely and lovingly from the early years communicated to their children that sex is a normal, healthy and wonderful experience, the basis of their parents' relationship, and the genesis of a new baby. Such alert and lucid parents who will and can answer their children's questions are regrettably in a minority, as survey after survey shows. But even such lucky children need more than the most informed parents can provide. Schools can provide more because they have teaching aids, libraries, skilled teachers and curriculum planning which can systematically provide a structure to meet the needs of the growing child.

But why should sexual knowledge be provided in the primary

school? Well, not *all* about sex, for this takes a lifetime to learn, or at least until adulthood is reached. No, sufficient to meet the needs of an enquiring mind, a developing body and later new relationships. Consider the needs of the following children *in terms of what they need to know*:

- a 3-year-old boy wanting to know why his baby sister hasn't got a sausage (a penis);
- a 4-year-old girl who asks why Daddy has nipples but no breasts;
- a 5-year-old boy who asks why girls don't pee standing up;
- two 6-year-olds, a boy and a girl, playing at 'mothers and fathers' in one of the bedrooms with no clothes on;
- a 7-year-old boy who over the family dinner table calls his sister 'a silly cunt';
- an 8-year-old girl early developer whose breasts are beginning to grow;
- a 9-year-old boy early developer who asks about pubic hair;
- a 10-year-old girl unprepared for the menarche who has her first period;
- an 11-year-old pubertal boy found trying to wash his bed-sheet after a nocturnal emission;
- a 12-year-old girl going out on her first date with a 16-year-old boy;
- two 13-year-old boys discovered engaging in mutual masturbation.[2]

All these situations are not uncommon. We are challenged by them to ask shall we simply reprimand, say 'Wait until you are older', or provide some intelligible information and support which will answer these children's needs? Beginning at least in the primary school years with a systematic understanding of sex would seem to be one important and sensible answer.

PART TWO
CHILDREN'S
SEXUAL EXPERIENCES

While Part One has been about children's knowledge (and ignorance) about sex, Part Two describes what children have actually experienced of sexuality. This section draws primarily on our most recent research with about 1000 first-year social science students in Australian universities, colleges of advanced education, technical and further education colleges, and apprenticeship schools. These male and female students were asked to fill in a lengthy questionnaire about what happened to them sexually as children before the age of 13, and also as young adolescents up to 16 years of age. The institutions sampled were from city and rural areas, involving a wide representation of social class, and the participants were on average 22 years, the majority of them aged 18 to 23 years of age.

What we report is based upon students' accounts of their sexual history during childhood and adolescence.[1] This reporting does not contain as much direct quotation from children as Part One, although we have included some statements from the previous study where they are relevant to the topic being examined.

Consequently in Chapter 8 we describe what children have experienced of the married life of their parents and how they look at the sex life of the ageing. In Chapter 9 we survey what kind of sexual embarrassments are experienced by children during family life. We then examine children's sexual experiences with other children in Chapter 10 and their sexual experiences with adults in Chapter 11. This latter chapter deals with the prevalence of child sexual abuse and how it affects the children concerned. Chapter 12 reports on sexual experiences of children with relatives, and Chapter 13 recounts the children's first direct sexual experiences and the ages at which they initially occurred.

In Part Two we describe research from other countries (principally the USA, Canada and Britain) on similar topics, so that a wider view of children's sexual experiences is given. It is not surprising that Australian students' sexual experiences when young are similar to those of their peers in other English-speaking countries.

8
PARENTS AND MARRIAGE

'My folks had a fantastic marriage. They did everything together, always happy, always supportive, never a cross word. My childhood was very settled and protected' (English boy, 15 years).

'All I can remember is the constant arguing, the rows and fights. I'd sometimes hear them shouting downstairs and I'd go to sleep with the pillows pulled over my ears' (American girl, 15 years).

Most children have a ringside seat on their parents' marriage, and are often acute observers of what goes on within the family. It is true that an increasing number of children experience broken marriages and may witness the decline and fall of a relationship. Some spend their entire childhood within a one-parent family and are not witness to a sexual relationship within marriage. But the vast majority of children do see from their ringside seats what kind of relationship their parents experience together.

Much of what the children see is not overtly sexual, but only marginally so, such as how (if at all) parents demonstrate affection for each other, how they discipline their children about sexual matters and what attitudes to sexuality they try to pass on to their children. To fill out this picture we used certain questions to see what children experience about the marriage which is the basis of their family life.

Looking back at their childhood 74% of these Australian students report being reared in an intact family. Thirteen per cent of them had parents who were separated or divorced, but most of these were marriages which lasted throughout childhood and were only broken after the children were in their late teens. A sizeable minority experienced a re-marriage, 7%

reporting growing up with a stepfather and 3% with a stepmother.

PERCEPTION OF UNHAPPY AND HAPPY MARRIAGES

We asked 'When you were twelve, how happy would you say your parents' marriage was at the time?' On a scale of unhappy to very happy we found 17% reported 'unhappy' and 'not very happy' marriages. Just over 80% reported 'somewhat happy' to 'very happy' marriages.

Asked to elaborate on what stresses were experienced in the marriages they observed at first hand, many reported a lack of energy exhibited by the mother in particular. Over 25% found their parents tense, nervous and worried, and some 12% had mothers who were often ill.

'There were times when it seemed we had no mother at all. She was in bed for long periods, or had a migraine. She couldn't cope. No wonder Dad was tense when he got home. We all had to help.'

Others reported fathers who drank heavily, and many mentioned both parents complaining about finances and having problems with relatives.

'I didn't know anything was wrong for a while but gradually my father began to sit up late with a bottle of whisky, just drinking and brooding. Then he'd go to bed drunk, wake up in the morning with a head[ache] and a foul temper. He'd go at us if we made any noise.'

One indicator to the children in a family is that even if parents have their differences, often described as arguments or rows, they may still demonstrate affection for each other by kissing, hugging each other or by holding hands. Some 32% reported they saw their parents kissing 'often' or 'very often'. If we add those who saw them kissing 'sometimes', the proportion increases to almost 60%. Some 16% said they never saw their parents kiss and 25% did so only rarely. These were the children who perceived their parents' marriage to be unhappy.

Hugging each other or holding hands as the demonstration of marital affection was reported by just over 40% of the students. Nearly 60% reported they never observed these affectionate activities.

'When we were young they used to smooch on the couch quite a lot, but I noticed later they'd just sit and watch TV and occasionally hold hands.'

'I never in my whole life saw my father touch my mother, kiss her or anything. They were always polite. I never thought it odd till later when I stayed with friends' families and saw much older parents being affectionate.'

Clearly many parents are inhibited about displaying their feelings in front of the children, what has been called 'a taboo on tenderness'. Fathers in particular were seen to be embarrassed at what might be thought of as unmanly behaviour, a curious idea since the male image is often thought of as aggressively sexy.

Regarding the sexual activity between parents or sexual intercourse, some 16% of our sample reported that they had seen or heard it when they were children. Of these most reported hearing through the bedroom wall or open windows in summer, since most parents try to ensure some privacy by keeping their bedroom door shut. One girl reports:

'I'd often hear funny noises from their bedroom. A lot of laughing and giggling and sometimes an odd kind of shout. It was very obvious at our beach house where there were very thin [wall] dividers.'

Nevertheless, some actually witnessed intercourse, even if it was by accident and momentary.

'I think I was 10 at the time and had just woken up in the morning and walked into their bedroom. I remember I thought it weird. All the bedclothes were on the floor, and there they were stark naked, Dad on top of Mum, moving up and down. He shouted to me "Get out" and I went and it was never referred to.'

Others were more systematically curious and yielded to a

voyeuristic temptation to observe through cracks in the door or chinks in the bedroom curtains. Most houses in Australia are one-level structures, so it is very easy to watch through windows at ground level, as this male student observes:

'I cottoned on what was happening when I was about 12 and could easily slip out into the garden and watch them. It was about then I began to masturbate.'

Although boys are more open in describing what they saw or heard of their parents' sexual activities, the girls were significantly more observant than the boys. And although most (84%) say they never saw or heard anything, many said they were aware that their parents did have sexual intercourse together.

The ages at which they say they first knew of their parents doing this is interesting. Seven per cent said they knew before the age of 7, but most were not aware of sexuality of this kind much before the age of 9 years. Another 56% of them said they knew of parents' sexual intercourse before they were 11. Some 30% knew about it in their young teens (11 to 13) and 7% at 14 years and older.

Despite their observations and a growing awareness that parents must have some kind of sexual joining in order to produce babies, children are still reluctant to accept the full sexuality of their parents. As we observed in the first chapter, there are many reasons why this should be so. So we have a curious situation where most people know and everyone pretends not to know. The sexuality of children exists but is denied wherever possible by parents. The sexuality of parents is known by children but denied wherever possible. And marriage itself, as we report later, is seen more as an economic or social unit than a sexual institution.

PERCEIVED PARENTAL ATTITUDES TO SEX

Families do teach about sex, not necessarily in terms of formal sexual knowledge, but rather in the attitudes to sexuality conveyed mainly by parents to their children. Rarely is there formal teaching on such matters but rather understanding comes from a long apprenticeship of watching, listening and observing often rather subtle signals or even body language from parents when certain sexual matters occur. Attitude formation results mainly from indirect learning, although some topics may be openly discussed in some families and the parents' views stated quite directly.

'I was never told by my parents not to do certain things but I knew what they thought about them. Like masturbation—I knew they disapproved but they never said anything.'

The students reported to us what they thought their parents felt about sexuality, conveyed both directly and indirectly. They also reported what they themselves now think about these matters. Consequently it is possible to judge how successfully an older generation is indoctrinating its young.

We found that parents and their children agree that 'Men often try to take advantage of women sexually', that 'Homosexual activity is abnormal' and that 'Sexual activity between members of a family is unhealthy'. This last reflects warnings and fears about incest conveyed by more than 90% of both mothers and fathers, attitudes agreed to by about 90% of their children. In these matters parental attitude formation looks as though it is highly successful.

But on two matters children are more progressive than their parents. While more than 50% of parents convey their negative judgment that 'Masturbation is unhealthy', about 85% of their children do not agree. In other words, most of their children regard masturbation as a normal and healthy sexual activity.

And while two-thirds of parents judge sex games among small children to be unhealthy, only about one-third of their children believe them to be so. As we shall see, the vast majority of students do report they had played sex games as children themselves and only a third felt such activities were unhealthy. So in these two rather important areas, masturbation and the sex games of children, parental attitude formation can be judged unsuccessful. In their turn, where the children grow up to become parents we can assume there will be more positive attitudes and greater tolerance, if not acceptance, of these sexual activities by children.

'Playing sex games with your playmates. Most kids do it. It's just natural curiosity and harmless. In fact it can do a lot of good if you don't know the differences between boys and girls. I won't tell my kids it's unhealthy.'

When we asked what sexual matters parents had punished, scolded or warned their children about, we found some very interesting responses. Top of the list was the saying of dirty words, which 80% of parents had punished, scolded or warned against. It is clear that 'dirty words' means sexual words, and sadly the use of the correct terms for the sex organs is often condemned. Doing something sexual on dates is also warned against by 40% of mothers, particularly to their daughters.

Not having clothes on in certain situations even within the home is condemned by more than a quarter of all parents, mothers in particular. About the same proportion condemn sex games with other children, and boys especially are warned not to look at sexy books and pictures, an edict disregarded by most boys in their teens who develop an insatiable curiosity.

'We used to look up pictures in the encyclopedias which showed pictures of men and women with their sexy bits showing. It was always when my parents were out because we knew they'd disapprove. My brothers and me tried to look up the dirty bits in the Bible but that was harder because we didn't know where to look.'

Mothers tend to warn both sexes about touching their own sex organs (17% mentioned this) but few warnings or scoldings are given about asking sexual questions despite the children's own stated reticence about making sexual enquiries of their parents. Most interesting of all is the low percentage giving direct warnings about masturbation, 10% of mothers and 7% of fathers. It may be that prohibiting touching of sex organs is a disguised way of tackling this habit. This illustrates the taboo nature of this topic even among parents, who nevertheless convey their disapproval of masturbation in other indirect ways. Why this should be so we deal with in more detail in the next chapter.

WHY PEOPLE GET MARRIED

'You gotta get married to have kids. Having kids is fun. You have birthdays and give presents. It's no fun on your own' (Australian girl, 9 years).

It is appropriate here to report on what we found in our first study on children's sexual thinking, concerning how children perceive the institution of marriage. We asked the question 'Why do people get married?' The evidence is, as we have already noted, that direct sexual reasons as the basis for marriage are rarely given. Even among teenagers, the 13- and 15-year-olds, only around 10% give sexual answers to this question. These rare replies include answers which indicate that people get married to have unlimited sex, to be able to kiss, neck, smooch or sleep together without restriction. Even important features such as sexual attraction are minimal; 'She thinks he's handsome and he thinks her pretty.' A typical example of this is given by a Swedish boy of 13 years:

'A man and woman are attracted to each other sexually. They want to live togther, sleep together, have children. So they get married and they can do it as much as they like.'

But very few, as we have noted, give such explicit sexual explanations.

More indirectly sexual is the reason given by most that people simply get married so they can have children. Remember that most children up to 9 years see no sexual activity in baby-making so they do not and cannot see marriage as a sexual union. Nor do many of them perceive that you can have children without getting married, as the following replies illustrate.

'So they can have babies. (Have you got to be married to have a baby?) Oh yes. The vicar says so, an' he won't Christian the baby if they're not married' (English girl, 7 years).

The logic is a little weak here but the general drift is that ex-nuptial babies are not acceptable in society, to clergymen or others.

'So they can have lots of children. (Have you got to be married to have babies?) Everyone's got to have a mother and a father. It's not right just to have a mother. (How do you mean?) 'Cause they put you in a home, and there isn't enough money. (Pause) It's not allowed' (Australian boy, 7 years).

This boy at the authoritarian stage of development obviously believes it is not only wrong, but also illegal, to have babies outside marriage.

More generally the need to have children comes out very strongly in most replies before the age of 11 years, and all sorts of reasons are given why people want them:

'They want children. (Why?) They grow up to look after their parents when they are old and can't work' (English boy, 11 years).
'To have children. (Why?) So they can be protected. (How do you mean?) Girls and ladies need to be protected' (English boy, 9 years).
'To have kids. (Why?) Well, it's lonesome on your own. Having kids around is better. You don't get lonely' (Australian girl, 9 years).
'Children. (Why?) Because two people can look after children better. (How do you mean?) When they're sick or need to be taken to school' (Canadian boy, 9 years).
'Having children. (Why?) It's in all of us. It just happens. (How do you mean?) We've all got to have children. It's in us' (American girl, 11 years).

The last 11-year-old is struggling to express some kind of biological urge, but cannot quite state it clearly. Teenagers in particular produce the necessity argument, not only biological drives but also the purpose of continuing the family name or the human race. So, why do people get married?

'Because of the children. (Why?) Because children help continue the family name and tradition. (How do you mean?) You want your family to go on. You don't want it to die out' (English boy, 13 years).
'It's to continue the human race. (How do you mean?) When you're married you have children and that's necessary for the world to go on living. It's important to keep on producing children to make up for those that die off' (Australian girl, 15 years).

Yet others at all age levels see the institution of marriage as the natural outcome of love. 'Because they love each other' was a reply given by more than 60% of the children, but only a few clarified this in terms of sexual love when asked. It was more a vaguely expressed idea of people liking each other, an extension of friendship, a little romanticised, rather than seen as a sexual union.

'They're in love. (How do you mean?) They like going to church and the flowers and the bridesmaids. (Is that why they get married?) Yes. They like doing the same things' (Canadian girl, 5 years).
'Because they love one another' (How do you mean?) They so like each other they want to be together all the time. They're good friends' (English girl, 7 years).
'Because of love. (How do you mean?) They're in love. They enjoy each other's company. He thinks her cute and she thinks he's handsome, so they get married' (American boy, 9 years).
'Love is what it's all about. (How do you mean?) They're very close and good friends. They like being together. It's good to have someone to share your worries and your whole life with' (Australian girl, 13 years).
'Because they're in love. (How do you mean?) You've got someone to depend on. It's good to have someone to depend on. You can't go on depending on your parents' (English boy, 15 years).

Some who saw love as a reason for marriage produced some realistic insights about the different kind of love involved.

'They're different from other loves, like loving your mother. (How do you mean?) Well, you leave your parents but when you are married you want to be together always' (American girl, 13 years).

131

'You marry to show your love and respect for another person. (How do you mean?) Having babies helps, it strengthens the bond between them. They've something to share' (Australian girl, 13 years).

Yet others, the few, show more social as well as sexual realism:

'A boy's got to show his responsibilities if he's got a girl pregnant. (How do you mean?) He'll marry her so the baby is OK, has a name' (Australian boy, 15 years).
'You don't have to marry. Not these days. If you have babies, unmarried mothers are more accepted in society' (Australian girl, 13 years).

These last remarks are echoed by many Swedish teenagers. In fact the different status of marriage as an institution in Scandinavia, and Sweden in particular, affected the Swedish responses quite drastically. Our Swedish colleagues who helped arrange the interviews in Stockholm pointed out that Sweden has abolished the term 'illegitimacy' and as a result numbers of ex-nuptial births, that is births outside marriage, are beginning to approach the totals of children born within marriage. In addition, in Sweden the number of de facto marriages has greatly increased. Swedish statisticians have forecast that within a short time half of Swedish 8-year-olds will live with a single parent and most of the other half will live with de facto parents. [1]

All this is not an expression of immorality in Sweden, for over 90% of the population are members of the Swedish Lutheran church. Laws such as those abolishing illegitimacy and recognising the validity of de facto marriages are simply an acceptance of long-established social practices. In the light of all these facts we might have been wiser not to have asked Swedish children 'Why do people get married?' but rather 'Why do a man and a woman want to live together?'

Among the English-speaking children there were two other reasons given for why people get married, both of them basically non-sexual. The first reason is shared by some Swedish children, namely economic saving.

'Two people can buy a home more quickly. And two can live cheaper than one, like sharing food and heating and such' (Australian boy, 13 years).

'It's not easy to move away from your parents, because they look after you. But a girl needs someone to take the place of her parents, to provide for her keep, buy her dresses and pay for holidays. So she marries' (English girl, 15 years).

But the other, the legalistic reason for marriage, was given by one in three of the English-speaking children but was given by only one in five of Swedish 15-year-olds, some of whom as ex-nuptial children had attended their parents' wedding! This apparently is quite a familiar pattern, that a couple may be in a de facto relationship for some years, have children, become convinced their union is reasonably permanent and then marry with their children in attendance. For the English-speaking children the legalistic reason is expressed in fairly conventional terms.

'It's right to get married if you want to live together. It makes your relationship more binding and you're more likely to stick together if you're legally married' (Canadian girl, 13 years).

'You should get married if you're going to have children. (Why?) So they can have a legal name and not be called bastards. It's something permanent the whole family can hang on to. It makes separation far less easy. If you have a row, you're not as likely to just walk out' (Australian boy, 15 years).

To sum up this section, few children see marriage directly as a sexual institution, although they do so indirectly by viewing it as an institutionalised expression of love or as a unit for begetting and rearing children. For some the reasons may be strictly legal or economic, although these are secondary considerations for the majority. Sexual reasons are often disguised, particularly in the teenage years when there is increasing reluctance to think of their parents as sexual beings. And because parents represent to children an older and ageing part of the population the next question is significant and relevant.

DO OLDER PEOPLE HAVE SEX?

In an early section of our interviews with children in five countries, we explored what they thought about old age. The first thing we confirmed was that young children were quite unrealistic about when a person is old, sometimes quoting 25 or 30 years as old. They only arrived at a realistic age of 60 or over by the age of 9 years, although Swedish children achieved this realistic view by 7 years. But many older children, including some teenagers, regarded their own parents as 'old', even when it appeared their parents were still in their 30s or 40s at the most.

The second discovery we made was that children aged 9 to 15 years in all countries, including Sweden, described old age in terms of sickness, weakness, deterioration, and negative features of this kind. Few voiced anything positive about old age, embracing what is basically a biological decline model.

This deteriorating picture of old age, as other research shows, is shared by later teenagers and young adults into their mid-twenties. It is not surprising therefore that the children and teenagers in our interviews made little or no allowance for sexuality in old age. Most teenagers, mainly girls, when they mentioned sexuality in old age pointed out the inability of older women to have babies. But both sexes made reference to the diminution, even extinction, of the sex urge in later years.

'You don't have the sex urge any more. (How do you mean?) Well, you don't want it. I suppose you've had as much of it as you want in your life. Women can't have babies anyway, so why do it?' (Australian boy, 15 years).

When we put together the picture of children beginning to classify their own parents as ageing, and the biological decline model of the aged, it is not surprising that many children either deny their parents' sexuality or see them as 'past it'. After all, they have produced children and after that, for some children, must lie sexual oblivion.

WHAT CHILDREN NEED TO KNOW ABOUT PARENTAL SEXUALITY, AND WHY

The family is the primary context for children's development, including their sexual development. Mothers and fathers serve as sexual models, as male and female ideals for their children. Obviously if the sexuality of parents is concealed, totally inhibited or denied by parents or their children, or by both, the potential for this natural process of sexual, as well as social, education may be destroyed.

Children need to see their parents showing tenderness to each other, demonstrations of affection, such as kissing, hugging or holding hands. Far too often we are inhibited by embarrassing thoughts such as 'not in front of the children', as though such tenderness is something to be hidden or to be ashamed of. These are needless and often damaging taboos parents may impose upon themselves, reflecting their own parents' inhibited attitudes. Yet children need to be aware that parents have needs and feelings which can be expressed.

There are, however, limits to what children may witness. We do not advocate that children or teenagers witness the act of sexual intercourse by their parents, although there is a minority view supporting this as the ultimate apex of sex education in the family. We do not support this for two main reasons. The first is that the sex act is an intensely personal act of love and commitment. Parents, as do their children, have a basic right to their privacy in these matters, just as they may wish certain acts of toiletry to be private. Few parents, for this reason alone, would accept their children being present to watch their sexual joining.

But more importantly the sex act can easily be misunderstood by children. For many it is puzzling, alarming, frightening and even perhaps violent, the very opposite of the picture of caring and tenderness that other aspects of family life may have built up. We do not subject children to situations in which they are made to feel bewildered, alarmed or frightened. And we know from media research that witnessing violence can have very destructive results on children's perceptions of themselves and of human relationships.[2]

Sexual modelling for children need not be complete. That is, it does not have to present the roles of both sexes in all their aspects. What children need to see and understand are the broad areas in which man and woman, husband and wife, complement each other and some of the ways their feelings of love and tenderness are communicated. It may well be that children will ask parents about love-making, especially if they are discussing how babies are made and the process of conception. Parents should be as honest and accurate about this as in all sexual matters and if they feel open enough, say something about their own love-making. What children do not understand can await another time or another explanation.

9
SEXUAL EMBARRASSMENTS IN THE FAMILY

'My parents were very touchy especially about anything to do with sex. The slightest thing seemed to embarrass them like leaving the top button of my blouse undone. We were never allowed in the bathroom together' (English girl, 15 years).

'Everything was open. No secrets in our house. If anything sexy came up it was treated naturally by my parents, like when my little sister dropped her pants at her birthday party, we all just laughed' (Australian boy, 15 years).

There are enormous differences between families about what may cause embarrassments, as the two teenagers above reveal. This covers a range from very tight control because of the vexation sexual happenings may cause, through to a more relaxed atmosphere where a sense of humour relieves possible tensions. Laughter, of course, may only be a superficial disguise for embarrassment but this is far better than over-controlled and over-sensitive reactions to what are, after all, fairly normal occurrences in family life.

We have already discussed nakedness and the wearing of clothes in Chapter 6, and the nervousness of many parents in talking about sex and the problems they experience in answering the basic questions of very young children. In this chapter we shall look in greater depth at the general picture of those sexual matters which seem to cause embarrassment to parents and siblings. Embarrassments may convey negative feelings such as shame and guilt, feelings which attach to sexuality and are the basis of sexual attitudes. On the other hand they may be useful social indicators, warnings of what conventionally is unacceptable behaviour, lessons which can be valuable experiences for the young.

What we report comes mainly from Australian students commenting on their childhood family experiences. These experiences are paralleled in other surveys done in America and Britain, and we shall include some of the comparative trends on such matters from these other countries. While there is quite a wide range of experiences between families, the picture of what seems to be the cause of anxieties and fears in most families seems to be a reasonably accurate one.

KISSING WITHIN THE FAMILY

The questions we asked centred upon the child's experience when 12 years of age, and it transpired that at that time 53% of mothers and 29% of fathers habitually kissed their children. Thirty-two per cent reported seeing their parents kissing each other often or very often, about 27% sometimes and nearly 40% rarely or never.

There are, however, certain occasions when kissing is more embarrassing than on others. Kissing goodbye is apparently natural for 82% of mothers and 62% of fathers. But kissing 'goodbye' on the lips is acceptable to only 37% of mothers and to about 20% of fathers. Clearly, kissing on the lips is perceived as more sexual than on the cheek and therefore is more restrained and limited. As examples of this, fathers are significantly more embarrassed in kissing sons, as are brothers with brothers and sisters with brothers, as one would expect.

'We were OK, we knew, to kiss our parents goodnight, a kind of peck on the cheek, but if it was on the lips it was too sexy' (Canadian boy, 13 years).
'We'd sometimes kiss goodbye when going away for a time. Not every day. But it was sort of a general hug and a kiss, not a smoochy kiss. We'd have been too embarrassed' (English girl, 13 years).

What is the basis for such feelings and the need for restraint? One reason is that kissing on the lips is regarded as sexual, whereas there are asexual kisses which are more symbolic tokens of affection. Another reason more compelling is that if lip kissing is sexual, then restraints must be imposed because of the possibilities of incest. For most parents, to be too demonstrative is to provide signals of sexuality which must not be encouraged between members of the same family, a taboo practised by most societies today. The fear of incest also lies behind the many other occurrences we report which cause family embarrassments.

SEEING CHILDREN NAKED OR IN UNDERWEAR

A question asked about this was 'Who would embarrass you if they were to see you naked?' Some 60% of Australian students say they would be embarrassed if their mother saw them and 73% if their father saw them naked. Daughters were particularly embarrassed if their father saw them naked. Similarly other sex siblings would be anxious if such an event occurred, especially sisters with brothers (72%) and brothers with sisters (about 50%).

The restrictions extended to being seen in their underwear, when the sex organs would be covered. Presumably the sex organs are still noticeable even if completely concealed by underclothes. Only 24% of them would be so embarrassed if mother saw them in their underwear, whereas about 50% would if it was their father who saw them. Daughters in particular felt this to be so with both parents. Again, siblings of the other sex would in particular be embarrassed if seen in their underwear; a sister seen by a brother, and a brother seen by a sister.

Emotions about being seen in underwear do not run quite so high as for being seen naked but they are still considerable, especially between other-sex persons in the family. Mother is the exception, presumably because children will have been accustomed to being seen by her when they are partially dressed, since supervision of dressing especially in the early years is part of the duties of motherhood. Fathers are not normally involved in such duties and so may be a greater source of embarrassment to their children.

'Looking back it was really a funny experience. Being caught in your undies was a worry. Not that anyone could see anything. I'd dash for a shirt and trousers if anyone came in I was so worried. Who taught me to do that?' (male student, 20 years).

Obviously it was the family, and primarily mother, who over a period of ten years or more conditioned her children to so behave. 'Modesty training' and incest fears combine to make such training very effective.

Although clothing may have little to do with it, how embarrassed are children taught to be if members of the family come into their bedroom without knocking? Only 28% of children felt anxiety if their mother did so, but 45% of them were worried if their fathers did, especially daughters. Other sex siblings were embarrassed by such an occurrence, especially brothers if sisters came in unannounced and sisters with brothers.

All kinds of reasons may be involved in such feelings, particularly the right to privacy and the strong feeling that someone might just barge in when not wanted – when one is dressing or doing something highly sensitive, included in which may be sexual habits. We shall discuss this later in this chapter when dealing with masturbation.

BATHROOM ETIQUETTE

Bedrooms are not the only areas in the home where privacy is expected. Bathrooms are also places where privacy is safeguarded. These often include toilets (or lavatories) and are therefore doubly the venue of embarrassment if someone enters when it is occupied. Even if there is no toilet included in a bathroom suite, those using a bathroom may be partially or totally disrobed, so that the same embarrassments at being seen naked or only in underwear can be experienced.

Forty per cent of our student sample said they would be embarrassed by their mother entering the bathroom if they were there, but 64% (girls in particular) said they would be if their fathers entered. Same-sex siblings entering a bathroom were not too much of a problem, but embarrassment was significantly high if a sister entered when a brother was there, and if a brother entered when a sister was there.

Again the sexual implications are clear, that there is the possibility of the sex organs being visible if a member of the family enters while someone is defecating, bathing or simply washing. Most mothers again seem exempt from causing embarrassment because of their lifelong more intimate association with their children's bodies. Fathers and siblings of the other sex are very potent causes of embarrassment, mainly for sexual reasons.

'We were always taught to lock the bathroom door and the loo [lavatory] specially. (Why?) Because it's supposed to be private and they're your private parts someone might see. (Who?) Well, you wouldn't want your father and brother to see them' (Australian girl, 15 years).

TELLING DIRTY JOKES

We asked to whom in the family, when they were twelve, they felt they could tell a dirty joke without being embarrassed. This was a euphemism for sexual stories which are very common in our culture as a semi-disguised outlet for sexual feelings. In some circles and with selected people these kinds of stories are acceptable ways of breaking the taboos on certain sexual topics.

It is of interest to know whom a child would feel confident to tell such a story or conversely be inhibited from telling. Just over 30% felt they could tell it to both mother and father. This means more than two-thirds of parents would feel inhibited because of the story's content, even if it were very funny.

In contrast more than two-thirds of the boys would not be embarrassed by telling a dirty story to a brother, but would be embarrassed telling one to a sister. Sisters' reactions to telling such a story to brothers are also negative.

Sexual stories are not only taboo breakers and an outlet for sexual feelings, but they also convey messages that the teller of them is sexually wise, knowledgeable and sophisticated. The telling of these stories about boys and girls engaged in sexual activities, honeymooners, parts of the human anatomy and many other matters, is all part of the pretence game about sex that both adults and children play. The fact that they are told mainly to one's own sex is a strong indication that this is so, and that the sexual prestige of the teller is involved. And the fact that most cannot tell them to parents is also a part of the pretence game, to keep from parents the fact that their children are more aware of sex than they care to think.

'I used to tell my brother some very dubious stories. (How do you mean?) You know, dirty ones. We'd laugh a lot and my sister would come in and say "What are you laughing at?" but we'd never tell her. (Why not?) It wouldn't be right to tell it to a girl. (Would you tell your father?) Oh no. He'd punish us, think we actually done it' (English boy, 15 years).

TELLING ABOUT SEXUAL EXPERIENCES

Within the family one would hope there would be those in whom children could confide about matters causing anxiety. Mothers in particular fulfil this role for their children because they are more accessible and possibly better listeners than fathers, although in these days of working mothers and shared domestic responsibilities it is to be hoped that fathers will be more accessible to children and develop child-rearing skills.

Children need to confide in someone about all kinds of experiences which trouble them, not least their sexual experiences. The truth, however, is that they may have little confidence in doing this with their parents without considerable embarrassment. The figures we show in later chapters relating to sex games with other children and also experiences of sexual abuse at the hands of adults reveal these misgivings. In fact, parents may be the last persons to whom their children would wish to confide their sexual experiences; only 16% of them say they would confide in their mothers and less than 7% in their fathers.

This is possibly the result of role conflict on the part of parents. They are the nurturants and care-givers for their children and as such foster affection and trust in them. At the same time parents are social trainers and disciplinarians seeking to ensure that children acquire standards, attitudes and behaviours consistent with those of the family. These, of course, tend to reflect the mores and folkways of the culture of which the family is a part. The nurturant and disciplinarian roles often come into conflict, especially where sexual matters are concerned. If, as often happens, a child violates a sexual rule, for example engaging in a sex game with another child when warned not to do so, it becomes difficult for the child to share anxieties about that experience to the person who laid down the rule in the first place.

It is significant that children are twice as likely to tell their sibling of the same sex about such an occurrence as to tell a parent. And children are four times as likely to tell a friend of the same sex about a sexual experience as to tell a parent. There is less risk in telling a sibling, and far less in telling a friend, simply because they are not disciplinarians. It is easier also, because it is less embarrassing, for a boy to confide in a boy, and a girl to confide in a girl about such matters.

'When I was 8 years old, I think, the boy next door and me were playing mothers and fathers. It was innocent at first then he stuck something up me and I started to bleed. I was scared to tell my mum 'cause I knew she would punish me. (What did you do?) I told my sister. Fortunately the bleeding stopped and no harm was done. But I really was scared' (Australian girl, 15 years).

Unfortunately siblings or peers will possess generally no more knowledge or wisdom than the children in need. Adult comfort as well as treatment may be required, but it is less likely to be asked for, the closer the relationship. The irony of such a situation is that the person with the closest relationship to the child, a parent, is the one least likely to be asked because of fear of reprimand or punishment. Here is an example which illustrates this dilemma from the child's point of view, one of the very few mentions of masturbation in all our interviews.

'I wakened up one night with the sheets all messy and I thought

I'd wet the bed. I knew the sheets were soiled, but my mother must have changed them that day because I got clean sheets. Soon after it happened again and then I started masturbating and I must have messed the sheets a lot. My dad tried to say something one day, I was about 12 then, but he was too embarrassed. And so was I. We never did discuss it and it was a terrible worry to me for years' (Australian boy, 15 years).

Masturbation is such a common problem that we deal with it in more detail, in the next section.

MASTURBATION ANXIETIES

Masturbation is such a taboo subject that little research has been possible, although the Kinsey surveys in America did indicate how widespread it is among adolescents and adults. Experts in sexuality, defining masturbation as the deliberate stimulation of one's own sex organs to achieve pleasure, state that it is so widespread that it must be considered normal behaviour in relieving sexual tensions or finding substitute sexual pleasure in the place of sexual intercourse. Masturbation is also the vehicle for often forbidden sexual fantasies.[1]

Various estimates have been made about the prevalence of masturbation, from Kinsey's 58% of women and 92% of men to a more recent survey, the Hite Report, which suggested that 82% of American women masturbated at some time. Another American survey found that this was not confined to the young and unmarried but that 70% of married men and 68% of married women masturbated.[2]

If these figures have any validity, and they appear to be well founded, why is it that more than half of our Australian parents indicate masturbation to be unhealthy and condemn it in their children? There are many reasons why this is so. First, there are traditional myths – myths long ago discredited – that masturbation is damaging to health and even sanity. Second, these are buttressed by the condemnation by certain religious groups of masturbation as a sinful act. Not all religions or denominations condemn it, but certain groups such as Roman

Catholics and Orthodox Jews still exercise a very strong negative influence. The third reason, however, is the most convincing, that in condemning masturbation in the young, even if parents practise it themselves, they are trying to deny or delay recognition of their children's sexuality. This appears to be the most basic reason and the continuation of myths, despite their obvious falseness, and the use of religious condemnation, are rationalisations by many adults used to minimise or conceal the fact that children are sexual. To accept masturbation in childhood is a recognition that children have a sexual aspect to their development.

All this negativism generates in children anxieties stimulated by the continuation of myths, religious or other condemnation, and the often unspoken but communicated disapproval of parents. Even though 85% of students in our Australian survey now accept masturbation as healthy, they nevertheless report early feelings of guilt and shame.

'I was taught not to touch my thing. It was naughty and dirty. No reasons were given, just dark hints that it was wrong.'
'My mother left me a medical dictionary, a very old one, with a bookmark in the page on self-abuse. It informed me that if I did it I'd go mad. It was all very frightening and I believed it at the time. I was 10 years old then.'
'My mother made one remark. "That's nasty. Don't let me see you do such a dirty thing again. If you do I'll tell your father." And I still remember that 15 years later.'
'I was taught by the nuns it was wrong and had to be confessed if I did it. Sometimes I was too scared to confess and then I felt very very guilty.'

Because masturbation is used often as a relief and comforting mechanism, negative and repressive comments tend to increase anxieties so that more relief and comfort is needed. Such negativisms are self-defeating since children, seeking relief from guilt and comfort in their discomfort, will tend to increase their masturbatory activities rather than decrease or terminate them.

When does masturbation begin in childhood? Some mild form of self-stimulation occurs in the very young as early as the second year of life, when children control their hands sufficiently to touch their own genitals and find it a source of pleasure. This often continues and increases through infancy and childhood but tends to increase more in the pubertal years. Male teenagers and young men are the most frequent masturbators in that they manipulate to orgasm, that is to ejaculation.

A survey conducted in Norway showed that up to one half of the children aged 5 to 7 years played with their genitals.[3] From 7 onwards, masturbation increases. In boys it is often stimulated in groups, one boy teaching others how to do it, whereas in girls it is more an isolated exploration or the result of accidental activity. To quote from the Norwegian survey

'When I was 10 years old my best friend Jim, who was two years older, showed me his penis and how to masturbate. We are still doing it together' (Norwegian boy, 14 years).
'It happened the first time when I was 9 and was climbing the rope in gymnastics. On my way down I had the rope between my legs and had my first orgasm' (Norwegian girl, 12 years).

Some boys, of course, may begin orgasmic masturbation as a solitary activity, linked closely with their first nocturnal emission. Very few girls, on the other hand, take part in group masturbation or learn it in this manner.

WHY CHILDREN NEED A POSITIVE NON-CONDEMNATORY CLIMATE IN THE FAMILY

As the evidence shows, there are great differences between families in their reactions to the sexual experiences of children. Yet even in the most supportive families few parents seem to feel comfortable with the many indications of their children's sexuality. As Floyd Martinson reports, children are more accustomed to hearing words like 'embarrassed', 'miserable', 'awkward', 'irritated', 'uncomfortable', 'afraid', 'confused', 'disturbed', 'distrustful', 'ashamed', 'depressed', 'repulsed', 'frustrated' and 'guilty', when sexual matters arise, all of which contribute to a negative picture of sexuality. These are more often heard than words such as 'proud', 'enjoyable', 'warm', 'comfortable', 'uninhibited', 'excited', 'beautiful' and 'accepted'.

Traditionally parents tend to emphasise the negative because of their fears about children's sexuality, of the criticisms of neighbours or of the wider community, and fears that if unrestrained their children will grow up to be sexual athletes, mature before their time. While some family embarrassments may be necessary to show children the social limits to certain kinds of behaviour, they should be minimised. What tends to be communicated to children is that sex generally is something only adults can experience and that even for grown-ups it is a secretive rather shameful activity about which little should be said or asked.

Children need to be raised in a more positive non-condemnatory family climate. In non-sexual matters we recognise their need for happy, fulfilling, rewarding and positive experiences which increase confidence year by year and provide the zest and enjoyment we associate with childhood. But in sexual matters children also need confidence not condemnation, and the slow and steady assurance that sexuality is a positive, healthy and beautiful experience. This is communicated by the ways in which members of the family demonstrate affection for each other, by the acceptance of various attitudes to dress and undress, and a minimal amount of fuss about the way family etiquette is observed.

This is important not only throughout childhood, but also for when children grow into maturity. For 'The child is father of the man', that is, all children are future parents who in turn will rear children and pass on attitudes, ideas and associations to do with sexuality to the next generation. There are signs that we are making sexual progress, in that embarrassments seem fewer than they were and children and students reveal they are more accepting of such matters as masturbation and children's sexual games than were their parents. But progress is slow, due to continuous pressures of the culture and society's traditional fears of sexuality, especially in children.

10
CHILDREN WITH OTHER CHILDREN: CURIOSITY AND EXPLORATION

'When we were about 7 my girl friend and I smelled each other between the legs. We were in the cubby house with boxes over our heads to hide our faces and heads turned towards the corner' (Australian female student, 20 years).

'When I was 9 I did a bit of kissing and cuddling with the girl next door, about the same age. We were fully dressed and pretended to be father and mother' (Australian male student, 21 years).

'We had mutual masturbation sessions. I was about 8 at the time, two or three times, I think with one or two male friends a year or two older. We just touched each other's genitals' (Australian male student, 21 years).

'We played at showing our genitals to each other, me and a boy, about 9 years. We kept our underwear on' (Australian female student, 18 years).

Playing sex games is a universal activity among children, although little has been known until now about how widely it is practised, at what ages it is most likely to happen and the types of play in which children are involved. Play is widely recognised as a method by which children explore ideas, release feelings, satisfy their curiosity and generally try to understand the situations they encounter. From early childhood through to adolescence play is an informal method of learning and exploration. Adults also play games, sometimes in fantasy and sometimes for real, often as imaginative ways to explore and to test the limits of what is socially acceptable behaviour.

It is not surprising that sex games are so common in child-hood, since so much sexual secrecy is practised by the adult world. We have already seen how children mythologise in order to explain how babies are made, what goes on during pregnancy and how babies are born. If they do not know the facts they invent them, to satisfy their curiosity and devise a satisfactory explanation. Such exploration is not confined to children's thinking. Its natural extension is to explore their own bodies and those of other children, especially the sex organs, about which they may be astonishingly ignorant throughout their childhood. Sometimes, despite adult prohibitions, children explore directly their own and other children's bodies. They are particularly curious about the organs of the other sex. The more prohibited such knowledge is, the more curious they become. Indeed the prohibitions and taboos associated with such activities are prime causes of children disguising their curiosity in the form of games. As we shall see, there is a vast variety of games children play to conceal their pursuit of sexual knowledge and experience.

The facts we now report, the first figures released in this hidden area, come from a section of our research where we asked students to describe any sexual experiences they had had before the age of 12 with other children. As in all other questions we did not define 'sexual' but rather asked them to report on what they thought to be any sexual experience. The answers give us for the first time a reasonably clear picture of the sexual experiences of children with other children.

HOW MANY HAVE SUCH SEXUAL EXPERIENCES?

Over 82% of the students reported they had had some kind of sexual experience with another person before the age of 12. Some of these were experiences with adults, the details of which we set out in the next chapter. But more than 60% of the total sample (64% of the male and 58% of the female respondents) reported sexual experiences with other children before they were 12 years of age. On average each of them described at least two such experiences.

In this respect boys appear to be slightly more sexually active than girls with other children, but the differences are not significant. Indeed, in some ways girls were equally active and just as curious as boys about sexuality.

'As a small child, I must have been 7 or 8, a girl friend and I would hold each other with no clothes on, pretending to be married. My mother caught us once and we stopped doing it' (female student, 19 years).

As the evidence indicates, the stereotype of boys being active and girls being passive sexually in their childhood activities is far from accurate.

'My sister who was 5 years old encouraged me to watch her urinate. I was a year younger. It was all part of playing mothers and fathers' (male student, 30 years).

But boys are initiators also as this male student reports.

'I once asked a primary school girl friend when I was 9 – she was 8 – to touch me on my genitals. We were playing cowboys and Indians, I think. Anyway I was tied up at the time. I had contrived that. She did not do as I asked but tickled me instead.'

AT WHAT AGES DO SUCH EXPERIENCES HAPPEN?

About 10% reported that these experiences occurred before the age of 6 years, just over 40% between 6 and 9 years, and nearly 50% between the ages of 10 and 12. Slightly more girls than boys had such experiences between 6 and 9 years, and slightly more boys than girls had them between 10 and 12 years.

It is interesting that there is such a considerable incidence of sexual activities among children in the years 6 to 12. These are the years put forward by Sigmund Freud as the years of sexual latency when, he suggested, children lose all interest in sex due to the repressive taboos enforced by adults. This may have been so in Viennese middle-class society towards the end of the nineteenth century, but it is clearly not the picture in late twentieth-century Australia.

It is true that Freud's society was probably more repressive sexually than our own, especially with children. But Freud's observations were based upon clinical cases of adult neuroses which came to his attention during analysis sessions, hardly a representative sample of the population. Clearly the picture is quite the opposite at the present day. The prohibitions and taboos are still with us, but children's sexual curiosity and play are widely expressed even if still concealed and disguised, as we have noted, under such titles as 'Mothers and Fathers' and even 'Cowboys and Indians'.

WHO ARE THE OTHER CHILDREN?

In most cases children tend to have sexual experiences or play sex games with children of about the same age. The age differences are usually no more than one or two years and occur in friendships of two children or groups of playmates of mixed ages.

Where there is a greater age difference the older child tends to take the initiative, and later when the younger becomes the older he or she in turn will tend to become the leader in such matters. In other words older children seem to induct younger ones into sexual activities, not in terms of initiation ceremonies but more like rites of passage for the age group, an expression of growing confidence, intimacy and willingness to explore.

There are the occasional experiences of a much older child with a younger child, where the younger is persuaded or cajoled, sometimes unwillingly, to participate in something sexual. For example

'When I was 9 my friend's older brother, in his teens, coerced us into playing a game, woven around our masturbating him' (female student, 22 years).

But this type of example is the exception. The most typical is that of children of nearly the same age, one or other taking the initiative but both agreeing to explore or engage in the activity suggested.

Most of the experiences described are in twosomes, during

a natural time of play, which usually occurs without the supervision of parents. Less than 10% of the incidents occur in groups of more than two, and where these happen they tend to be in mixed groups or solely male groups. Groups of girls do not appear to be interested in sexual exploration, although this does happen in some girl twosomes.

Boy and girl twosomes are the most common but with 80% of the boys playing with girls and 62% of the girls playing with boys. More girls play with girls (26%) than boys with boys (12%) where sexual experiences occur. In other words the vast majority are in heterosexual twosomes, children showing considerable curiosity about the sex organs of the other sex. The minority are homosexual twosomes, the greater number of these being feminine twosomes.

RELATIONSHIP TO OTHER CHILDREN

Only an insignificant number of cases were of children sharing a sexual experience with a child who was a stranger. This is not surprising since most children mix with other children who are known, in kindergarten, school, Cubs or Brownies, or neighbourhood playgroup meetings. The large majority of sexual experiences in childhood occur with other children who are friends, distant relatives such as cousins, or closer relatives such as brothers or sisters, that is, siblings.

About two-thirds of these experiences are with friends and, as we have seen, those of roughly the same age group, or a single friend of the other sex. They are not sought out for specifically sexual reasons but rather the sexual activities tend to arise incidentally in the course of other kinds of play.

'We were playing in our garage with a box of dressing-up clothes. The girl next door and me. We were about 8 or 9 years old. When we took our clothes off to get dressed up we looked at each other all over. It happened a few times and we began to touch the sex parts. It was all very innocent' (male student, 19 years).

Cousins who live nearby are often play companions. Distant

cousins may stay overnight or longer and these are opportunities for sexual experiences to occur. About 11% of our student sample reported such happenings.

'She was a girl cousin who came to stay a week. We were about the same age, about 9, and I remember we got into bed together and had a kiss and a cuddle. My mother moved me while I was asleep to my own bed' (male student, 30 years).

'A cousin, a boy, came to stay with us. When no one was home he took out his penis and showed it to me. I was scared to touch it but he touched me between the legs. It was naughty I knew, but it felt nice. I was 11 and I think he was 12' (female student, 24 years).

Sexual experiences between siblings will be reported more fully in the next chapter dealing with children's sexual experiences within the family. However, we report here that 11% of those who describe sexual experiences with other children before the age of 12 describe them as occurring with siblings. This is about 7% of the total sample. The vast majority of these are a brother and sister together, that is, involve some kind of heterosexual exploration or game. There are more sister with sister experiences than there are brother with brother.

We prefer to call these intra-family sex experiences with siblings rather than use the more emotive word 'incest'. The taboos on incest are very strong in our society, although children become aware of them only gradually during childhood. It is perfectly natural for siblings when enjoying the nighttime bath together to see, comment on and explore each other's sex organs, especially if left unsupervised even for a few minutes. Holidays at the beach and camping expeditions, playing at home when parents are absent, all present opportunities for sexual exploration and the satisfying of curiosity.

'It happened every bath time over about three years. My sister showed her sex organs to me and I showed her mine. I was 7 and my sister was 4, I think' (male student, 21 years).

'My brother and I would play at being mothers and fathers. When they weren't home we'd go to bed fully clothed and roll about on top of each other. It was a bit of a giggle really' (female student, 19 years).

'When we were about 5 and 6 we'd play at being babies. I remember sprinkling some cleaning powder on my sister's vulva and putting a nappy on her' (male student, 28 years).

The majority of such experiences between siblings involve mainly the showing of sex organs to each other, the occasional touching of the sex organs, and perhaps a certain amount of sexual fondling.

The more overt and sophisticated sexual experience is rather rare. One female student states that at the age of 10 she persuaded her younger brother to attempt intercourse with her, but the attempt was apparently unsuccessful. And on one occasion they painted each other's genitals with house paint. What the consequences were when the paint dried we are not told.

WHAT RANGE OF SEXUAL EXPERIENCES ARE INVOLVED BETWEEN CHILDREN

From the accounts already given it will be seen that there is a very wide range of sexual experiences involved when children are active with other children. But it is not only the range of activity, but what is most likely to happen, that concerns most parents. To help get a clearer overall picture we classified the experiences described by students in an ascending order of intimacy, which we report below.

Of the 60% describing sexual experiences with other children before the age of 12

66% report an invitation to do something sexual
67% report kissing and hugging in a sexual way
78% report other child exhibiting sex organ
68% report child exhibiting sex organ to other child
62% report being fondled in a sexual way
56% report fondling other child in a sexual way
58% report other child touching sex organ
53% report child touching other child's sex organ.

Exhibitionism was the most commonly reported behaviour, but the figures for other activities are also quite high.

Of the remaining categories of sexual activities, 'almost sexual intercourse without penetration' was reported in 18% of cases. These cases, eighty-six of them out of a total of almost one thousand students, included mutual masturbation and activities often called 'genital apposition', the rubbing of the sex organs together to achieve sexual excitement.

In ten cases there is a report of intercourse or attempted intercourse, mainly by older children in the 10-12 age group. One case of oral sex was reported and one case of pretending to be breast fed. But overall, the picture is one of playful curiosity and a mutual exploration of sexuality, not of the sexual reproduction activities or sexual pleasures of mature adults.

WHAT KIND OF SEX GAMES?

We have already commented that children's sexual games are ways of disguising activities known to be prohibited. This disguise is probably largely unconscious, sexual ideas often occurring as an incidental feature. Indeed, the players may be innocent of any sexual motive, until one member of the duo or larger group introduces a sexual theme as the play develops. Some games, however, are quite blatantly sexual but presumably by their disguise still provide some kind of avoidance of guilt on the part of the players.

We shall look at the first type of game where sex is incidental to the major theme, compared with the second type where sex is the main preoccupation.

Cowboys and Indians

Several students describe playing this game but there are many variations. The major theme is hunting or being hunted, with often a minor theme of a captured squaw or cowgirl, who may be played by a boy or a girl. A rescue is attempted and some kind of sexual excitement is experienced at the idea of bondage or winning the love of the squaw or cowgirl. Such fantasies involve kissing, hugging and fondling but these are only incidental to the main action.

War games

These also provide major themes of conflict and violence between opposing sides and male soldiers being captured. The sub-theme is of a sympathetic girl who will comfort, free or demonstrate some affection for the prisoner. This may involve body contact, the idea of bondage or simulated torture, all of which may include seduction of one sex by the other, but more in terms of fondling than intercourse.

Mothers and fathers

This also is a game with many variations, some more overtly sexual than others. Themes include having a tea party, discussing the children, dressing for dinner and undressing for bed. Children explore the roles of mothers and fathers in this type of play so it is not surprising that the secret sex roles of parents are also the subject for playful investigation. A more sexual theme within this may be 'Getting married' which may contain an innocent reconstruction of a wedding but may also clumsily try to simulate what is thought to be sexual union as its consummation.

Doctors and Nurses

This provides a more overt setting for body examinations, including the sex organs, since medical situations on a doctor's couch or in a hospital can be fantasised. This may take the form of a doctor or a nurse examining patients, telling them to take off their clothes or open their legs or adopt similar postures. Alternatively doctors and nurses together may become amorous, as in so many medical television soap operas.

Drunks and Barmaids

This was a game mentioned by several students as one they played as teenage children. Such scenes are also stimulated by television, the sexy barmaid and the befuddled drinker providing an excuse for a great deal of fondling and groping. Another game with erotic potential, usually for older children, is 'Photographers and Models', where the subject is usually a girl taught to pose by the male photographer who will have all kinds of physical contacts with her, possibly with sexual suggestions included.

Masturbation games

These are played generally by boys competing with each other to see who can come first or have the biggest spurt when ejaculating. Usually such games begin by an experienced masturbator teaching an inexperienced one how to do it. Such activities may occur when boys sleep together either in the same bedroom or in dormitory situations.

THE USE OF THREATS OR FORCE BETWEEN CHILDREN

When sexual experiences occur, whether in the form of direct contact or disguised in sex games, they may be initiated by a boy or a girl or both. The more important question to ask perhaps is whether one child coerces another in some way by the use of force or by threatening the use of force.

Only 18% of those describing sexual incidents with other children report threats of this kind being made and more than half of these qualified it with the words 'a little'. The other 82% said they had not been threatened, and 93% said they had not threatened the other children in attempting to gain their co-operation. All this indicates that the vast majority of these happenings are mutually agreed, or once begun are gone along with by the younger partner, since they may stimulate or satisfy sexual curiosity.

WHAT KIND OF REACTION OCCURS?

Yet another important question to ask is what were the reactions of children to these sexual experiences once they had occurred. When asked whether they had felt fear, shock, surprise, interest or pleasure, only 14% reported negative feelings. Another 15% reported surprise, and 70% said they had found the experience interesting or pleasurable. This is in direct contrast to their reactions to sexual experiences with an adult, which we report in the next chapter. However, of those who found their sex experiences with other children negative, girls outnumber boys by four to one. In other words, girls are more vulnerable than boys in feeling the negative effects of such experiences. This was confirmed when we asked what each student felt retrospectively looking back on the experience. Only 15% felt the experiences described to be negative but again girls far outnumbered boys in these reactions. But most of them thinking back concluded that the experience was positive (49%) or a neutral event (36%).

TELLING AND CONFIDING ABOUT SUCH EXPERIENCES

Since childhood sexual activities are so often tinged with guilt, it was useful to discover whether children told anyone, or felt able to tell anyone, about sex experiences with other children. And if so, in whom would they feel comfortable confiding?

About 63% of those who had such experiences told no one, indeed did not feel the need to tell anyone. Just over 20% confided in a friend, boys doing so significantly more than girls, the friend usually being of the same sex. About 8% told a sibling, but only 6% told their mothers and 2% their fathers. These small percentages who told their parents are not surprising, since sexual activities of any kind are recognised by children as tabooed areas by adults. Parents convey their vetos, their dislikes and their warnings, often indirectly, about sexual matters in general and overt exploration in particular.

More specifically, when the students were asked what they expected the reactions of their parents would have been if they had told them about their sexual experiences with other children, most forecast only negative responses. More than half said their parents would have been angry with them and the other child involved, and only about a quarter felt parents would have been supportive of them. These anticipated negative reactions were about the same for both mother and father. From other comments about how children view their parents as sexual disciplinarians we know that they would expect disapproval, condemnation or punishment of some kind if they told about such incidents. This also was the basis for the children's expectations and hesitations in telling their parents about any adult sexual abuse, as we describe in the next chapter.

Despite this inhibition on the part of children, some 2% of the incidents described were reported through their parents to officials. There were twenty-two cases where incidents were reported to police, medical authorities, a priest, children's officers and teachers (the last two groups being the more numerous). It appears that such reports were made when children were so hurt or distressed by an experience that they felt they had to tell, both as an expression of fears and a desire that such events should not happen again. The other side of this is that more than 90% of the experiences were not reported to the adult world. Even if frightened or fearful, children may be even more frightened to confide in any adult what has happened.

DEALING WITH SEXUAL EXPERIENCES BETWEEN CHILDREN

It must be said frankly that this area of sexuality is not an easy one for parents or teachers to handle, either before such experiences occur or once they have become known. As in other areas, there is a role conflict between being modesty trainers, disciplinarians and guardians of social norms and being the confidants, supporters and comforters of the young. This potential conflict is not of the children's making but is implicit in the social roles expected of adults in child rearing. However, such conflicts may be alleviated if not removed by a more understanding approach to childhood sexuality on the part of parents, teachers and other adults involved with children. It is the responsibility of adults to come to terms with the needs of children and to develop attitudes and strategies to deal with their needs adequately and positively. Condemnation and repressive measures are usually the resort of frightened or embarrassed adults who know of no other ways of dealing with the sexual experiences of children with other children.

Recognise the basis of children's sexual explorations

Such experiences cannot be dismissed as evil manifestations or the expression of original sin. To place them in such a moral context is inappropriate, since children are slow to develop moral ideas. Sexual values only become evident and possible at a later stage of childhood when more abstract thinking becomes feasible.

There is nothing immoral or wicked about the desire to explore reality, which all children reveal is basic to their nature from a very early age. Children explore sexuality in their own bodies, and in the bodies of others, just as they explore their gardens, toys, houses, play areas and a whole range of ideas with which the adult world presents them. Admittedly there are dangers from which we try to protect children. Hot stoves are to be avoided, so are sharp instruments, sudden falls and other environmental dangers. But we do not try to restrict exploration simply because these dangers exist, for this is how children learn.

The bases of sexual exploration lie in a natural curiosity which is the most effective drive to learning. Such curiosity is greater if sexuality has been kept secret, if sexual enquiries and questions are sidestepped or if misinformation is deliberately given. When a small boy points to his penis and says 'What is it?' he may be told 'You shouldn't ask such a question', 'I'll tell you later when you are old enough to understand' or 'That's your willie.' All these replies convey evasion and reluctance. A much healthier and educative approach is to call it by its correct name, a penis, and to answer straightforwardly such follow-up questions as 'What's it for?' and 'Why hasn't my sister got one?'

We have seen that curiosity about the sex organs is the reason for most of the sexual explorations and sex games children play. Exhibiting a sex organ to another child, and touching and fondling it, are the major purpose in such exploration. All this is stimulated much more when prohibitions are made. If accepted as a natural and normal mode of enquiry by children their search will not become obsessive, which is what many adults fear. It becomes a natural and incidental activity just like any other playful exploratory experience.

Accept children's sexual play as normal

Because of their own restrictive upbringing, many adults have difficulties with this idea. Their own guilt feelings and negativisms about sex accumulated during childhood and adolescence may make it difficult to accept that most of children's sexual explorations with other children are normal.

By normal we mean that if most people or most children practise such behaviour it is or becomes 'the norm', that is the acceptable standard or performance of a person. The evidence we have presented indicates that about two-thirds of children engage in sexual exploration with other children. In the same way we are beginning to accept masturbation as normal, since the evidence shows that most people, of both sexes, use it as a means of sexual relief or fantasy at some time in their lives.

Another way of defining something as normal is not only by reference to its known universality but to the fact that it is natural. Sexual curiosity is not artificial; in most cases it is not something which is imposed but arises from the child's need to know and understand reality.

What is encouraging is the evidence from our study. Students reporting on their sexual experiences as children felt their parents condemned sex games among children as unhealthy. But more than two-thirds of the students themselves accepted them as normal and natural activities from which they derived benefit. In the same way the students accept masturbation, including masturbation games, as normal and natural. Attitudes to such matters are obviously undergoing a change towards greater acceptance of what was once thought to be sinful and even abnormal. This makes it easier for future generations of parents to become more positive and accepting of such matters.

Judge when children's sexual play is abnormal

There are some children's experiences with other children which have to be recognised as abnormal, that is, unacceptable. Experiences which hurt children physically or are frightening to them, causing fears, outbreaks of crying and nervous reactions, cannot be accepted in any sense as normal. These kinds of happenings are mercifully in a minority when children are with other children, but they do happen and children should be protected from them.

Where children are coerced to do something sexual against their will by another, possibly older, child and perhaps bullied into acquiescence, different kinds of consequences occur. They may range from discomfort to outright pain. A child may object to being fondled, or being made to touch another's sex organ. We can cite two examples, one of a girl made to perform oral sex on an older boy, and another of a girl inserting a bottle in another girl's vagina 'to see if it fits', causing severe bruising and bleeding.

Rather than subject mystified children to vague or specifically frightening warnings about this kind of possible incident, we suggest that the 'No', 'Go', 'Tell' preventive programs about child sexual abuse (which we review in the next chapter) not be confined to what adults can do to children. What is taught may well apply to what other children may do.

Briefly, children should be taught to say 'No' to anything anyone wants to do with their bodies which makes them feel uncomfortable, unsafe or frightened. They should 'Go', that is, leave the offending person and place where the experience happens and get to a place or person with whom they feel safe.

And they should 'Tell' some adult, preferably a parent, if they feel frightened and if they fear it may happen again. This telling, of course, depends on the trust built up between parent and child and the child having an expectation of being understood and comforted rather than condemned or punished.

These abnormal events must, however, not be allowed to dominate adults' thinking about children's sexual explorations with other children, the vast majority of which are perfectly normal and acceptable within the allowed limits of natural social learning.

11
CHILDREN WITH ADULTS:
CHILD SEXUAL ABUSE

'There was a close family friend, a man, who used to come to our house. He was a member of my father's church. He'd fondle me in a manner I didn't like. When I told my parents I was smacked and told I was sinful with a filthy mind, and that the man in question was a Christian so it couldn't possibly be true. I was about 8 at the time. I never confided in my parents again' (Australian female student, 20 years).

'A male in his 40s tried to molest me in a primary school toilet, tried to touch my penis when I was weeing. I was allowed to leave after he'd exposed himself and I think masturbated. I must have been no older than 6' (Australian male student, 19 years).

While the majority of children do not have such experiences, our study present the first Australian figures on this subject. We found that 28% of Australian girls report some kind of sexual exploitation by an older person, and 9% of Australian boys so report. That amounts to between one in three and one in four of girls and about one in eleven boys. More than 90% of such incidents are perpetrated by men. These figures are sufficiently large to cause concern and they are not confined to Australia. Similar findings are reported in studies in America, Canada and Britain.[1] These experiences of children with adults are called by several names such as exploitation, victimisation, molestation or abuse. In this discussion we use the most widely used term, child sexual abuse.

WHAT IS CHILD SEXUAL ABUSE?

Children are particularly vulnerable to adults who approach them for the purpose of sexual activity. Adults are to most children powerful authoritarian figures who require obedience. For many children these adults are to be believed, trusted, obeyed, and their suggestions or directives are to be followed. Children throughout their growing years are taught to trust the adult world and they are naturally dependent upon those much older than themselves.

Child sexual abuse occurs when an adult takes advantage of a trusting child and persuades or tries to persuade that child to do something sexual. This is an abuse of adult power because it is an exploitation of the trust and respect children are trained to demonstrate to their elders. For this reason the most accurate way of defining child sexual abuse is by estimating the age difference between a child and the adult concerned.

In this study we classify these age differences into three categories. First, there are cases where a child 12 years of age or under has some sexual experience with an adult who is 19 or more, making an age difference of at least seven years, and usually much more, where the sex abuser is clearly regarded as an adult. The second category is where a child 12 years or under is abused by an adult who may be under 19 but is at least five years older than the child. Thus an 8-year-old girl may be exploited by a 14-year-old boy, because she will regard him as grown-up. Many younger children regard teenagers in this light. The third category of age difference is where an adolescent is aged 13 to 16 years and is exploited by someone at least ten years older. Since in most states 16 is the 'age of consent' for sexual activity we have not gone beyond that age, and by using a minimum of a ten-year age difference we have eliminated what could be regarded as sex mutually agreed upon by two teenagers. While such mutually agreed activity may have some elements of exploitation it tends to be more an activity between those of the same age group.

All the three age differences discussed above show the relative powerlessness of the young. This is in sharp contrast to the partners who wish to use them sexually, who are older and more powerful, physically and psychologically, than the children being used.

'This uncle of mine would put me on his knee and pet me when I was about 10. He'd put his hand up my pants and try to touch me. I knew it was wrong. I didn't feel nice. But once he'd started I had to let him. He was my uncle' (Australian female student, 24 years).

WHAT SORT OF THINGS HAPPEN?

There are many myths about child sexual abuse, many people believing that it can only be defined in terms of forcible sexual intercourse or rape. Sexual intercourse, however, shows a small incidence in child sexual abuse; about 5% of the 28% of Australian girls reporting abuse had had experiences of such an extreme, traumatic nature. In order to see the picture with some accuracy we asked our subjects to signify if they had been asked to do something sexual by an adult person. The sexual activities we asked them to indicate were:

- an invitation to do something sexual;
- being hugged in a sexual way;
- the adult showing genitals to the child;
- the adult getting the child to show genitals;
- the adult fondling the child sexually;
- the adult getting the child to fondle him/her sexually;
- the adult touching child's genitals;
- the adult getting the child to fondle adult genitals;
- simulated intercourse without penetration;
- sexual intercourse.

All ten of these categories can be described as child sexual abuse. Some subjects reported a number of them, while some reported only one, that is the one considered the most 'serious'. Fondling and touching sometimes included masturbation or mutual masturbation.

The picture which emerges for Australian girls is that most of them who reported sexual experience mentioned some sexual fondling and the touching of genitals, child's or adult's, together with sexual exhibitionism by the older partner, that is, the display of genitals. These make up two-thirds of the sexual happenings experienced by girls, with 10% experiencing simulated intercourse, sometimes including oral sex or genital apposition without penetration, and 5% actual or attempted intercourse. (These, of course, are percentages of the one in three or four girls reporting child sexual abuse, so that the true figure of forced sexual intercourse is 1.4% of all girls, namely about fourteen in every thousand.) These figures are still disturbing, but if we are trying to picture a typical child sexual abuse occurrence it is far more likely to involve, for girls, sexual exhibitionism, sexual hugging or sexual fondling.

Boys are more likely to experience the touching of their genitals (43%), relatively few (10%) being fondled sexually or experiencing exhibitionism. Some six boys report anal intercourse accomplished or attempted by a male offender. Again, while disturbing, the figure in the total of male students reporting this is less than 1%.

While we can disprove the myth that the typical child sexual abuse is one of intercourse or attempted intercourse, the picture remains a disquieting one. As we shall report later, exhibitionism, fondling sexually or touching of genitals is quite frightening and certainly confusing to children who experience them, especially girls.

AT WHAT AGE ARE CHILDREN AT GREATEST RISK?

There is a common assumption that the young are more vulnerable and open to sexual abuse when they are in their teenage years, that is, when their pubertal and sexual characteristics are more obvious. The facts are otherwise.

The average age of children experiencing child sexual abuse in Australia is for girls 9.8 years and for boys 10.3 years. Most will not have developed sufficiently by that time to be called adolescent. But a closer examination of the figures for each age group shows a very wide spread across all age groups. The highest incidence of sexual abuse of girls occurs when they are

167

aged under 12 years, with a partner 19 years or older. The next highest for girls is when they are under 12 years with a partner five years or more older than themselves. Only 27 girls out of 603 (4.5%) report being sexually abused at between 13 and 16 years by a partner ten years older than themselves. Where boys are concerned, the highest incidence is for those aged under 12 years with a partner five years older than themselves. The next highest is when aged under 12 years with someone 19 years or older.

What these figures indicate is that the most dangerous years for the young in terms of sexual abuse are from 8 to 11 years, although some cases, especially with girls, do occur earlier. Some 28% of the girls reporting sexual abuse said it occurred when they were between 7 and 9 years, and for some 15% it was between 4 and 6 years. The figures are similar for boys in these age groups. So while there is some sexual abuse of those in the adolescent years from 13 to 16, these are certainly not the years when the young are at greatest risk.

WHO ARE THE ABUSERS?

The common assumption made is that abusers tend to be older men in their fifties or sixties and that they are strangers to the children. Such a stereotype called 'the stranger danger' typifies the abuser luring a child into his car or home by the promise of rewards such as lollies or money. Apart from the fact that over 90% of abusers are male, this common assumption is wildly erroneous.

Take the age of abusers, for example. The average age of abusers of girls is 31 years of age, far below the age stereotype of 'the dirty old man'. The average age of abusers of boys is even younger at 23 years. These figures are based upon estimates of students looking back at their experiences and are therefore to be taken broadly. Even so, they are the only indicators we have which appear to be reasonably accurate. In general, then, abusers tend to be in their twenties to early thirties seeking out mainly children aged 8 to 11 years. Looking at the more than nine out of ten abusers who are male, we see that the older males seek from girls some kind of heterosexual experience and the younger males seek some kind of homosexual experience from boys.

We have no direct evidence of the kind of personality common to abusers, but anecdotal evidence from many victims of child sexual abuse give us some clues.[2] Far from being dominant, aggressive and cruel people, abusers tend to be inadequate, often timid, personalities who cannot cope with adult sexual relationships. They find children to be more malleable and easier to deal with sexually because they are more docile and obedient. The fact that only a small number of abusers seek intercourse indicates their sexual inadequacies. They tend to be satisfied with displaying their genitals or manipulating them, using children more for sexual stimulation rather than consummators of the full sexual act.

Where 'stranger danger' is concerned, of those reporting sexual abuse by an older partner in Australia 26% say it was with a stranger. By contrast, some 74% of those experiencing child sexual abuse report it having occurred with someone known to them. These were friends or acquaintances, friends of parents or members of their own families. Relatives, details of which we present in the next chapter, make up 35% of girls' experiences and 18% of boys'. Cousins and nephews or nieces, uncles and aunts, brothers and sisters, fathers and stepfathers, as well as grandfathers, are among the abusers described under 'relatives'. So in many ways the sexual dangers children are open to are not so much outside but inside the family circle, especially when friends or acquaintances of the child's parents are included.

A question to ask about child sexual abusers is why is there such a preponderance of men? There is no direct evidence to answer this question and we can only provide a few tentative answers. First there is the cultural emphasis upon the traditional sexual aggressiveness of the male as hunter and initiator of the sexual act. Although it can be argued that the sex drive is equally strong in men and women, the culture certainly stimulates a more active sexual role on the part of men.

A second cultural emphasis is upon male dominance generally, not only in sexual terms, but also in terms of power,

169

authority and the status of being head of the household. There is evidence where intra-familial sexual abuse is concerned that a patriarchal father is more likely to sexually abuse his daughter. Applied in a wider sense it can be argued that men are used to being obeyed, especially by women, and so sexual abuse of children is an extension of their dominating roles.

A third feature of our culture is the strong association of women not only with child-bearing but with child-rearing. The view has been advanced that the very closeness of physical nurturing, including breast feeding, toilet training, cleaning and bathing of children, inhibits a mother from thinking of sexual intimacy with the young to satisfy her own adult sexual needs. The physical satisfactions involved in these nurturing activities provide both a different kind of intimacy and at the same time may act as an inhibitor of overt sexual activity with the young of either sex. In other words, women learn much earlier and more effectively to distinguish between sexual and non-sexual forms of affection.

It may be argued that as men accept a more equal and less dominating role in society their proneness to be sexual abusers may diminish. And as men participate more in child-rearing and accept the more intimate aspects of raising children they may experience the inhibitions currently experienced by women.

THE USE OF FORCE IN CHILD SEXUAL ABUSE

Many case histories of child sexual abuse reveal that children may be persuaded, cajoled and induced to accept sexual activity by rewards or the promise of rewards. Even though they may feel it to be wrong, children will sometimes yield to such blandishments and appear to co-operate in some kind of sexual activity with such an adult. What is more disturbing, however, is the use of force or the threat of force in persuading a child, which makes the experience even more frightening and traumatic.

When asked whether force or the threat of force was used in their experiences of sexual abuse by older partners, 58% of Australian girls in our student survey reported this happening, but only 14% of the Australian boys. This illustrates the dominating nature of the male offender as the seeker of hetero-sexual experiences and the vulnerability of girls to this kind of threat. Students reported the threat of violence such as punish-ment by spanking or being hurt in some way, but often the threats were more subtle than the outright use of force. In general, it is probable that boys are less intimidated by threats, or thought to be so, and are offered alternative inducements to persuade them to co-operate. This certainly seems to be the case from the boys reporting their experiences.

One common persuasive ploy used by abusers, especially after the event and especially where the offender is known to the child, is the attempt to pledge the child to secrecy. 'This is our little secret' is often accompanied by some indications of the dire consequences for the child or the family if the secret is revealed. Obviously this kind of promise is strengthened if the child fears, however vaguely, all kinds of punishments or other consequences. So in addition to the trauma of the experience itself, children are often given a double burden of guilt and dishonesty. They report being ashamed by the need to conceal and behave in a furtive underhand manner.

WHAT EFFECT HAS SEXUAL ABUSE ON CHILDREN?

In contrast to children's sexual experiences with other children, which provoke reactions of surprise, interest or pleasure, their sexual experiences with adults are much more negative. Asked how they felt at the time, 68% of girls reported very negative reactions of fear or shock, during and immediately after the experience, while 30% of boys reported similar negative feel-ings. Asked how they felt at the time of interview, ten years or more later, 71% of the girls said they still regarded their experience as negative and disturbing while about 32% of the boys felt so. The evidence is that far from time being the great healer the significance of the occurrence of sex with an adult becomes more apparent as a person grows older and feelings of repulsion may in fact increase.

Children involved in such incidents appear to be more disturbed when the difference in age between the child and

171

the abuser is greater – that is, an 8-year-old will be less disturbed after an experience with a 13-year-old than a 10-year-old with an older person in their twenties or thirties. This is not surprising, since children will perceive a greater incongruity of the experience the wider the age gap becomes. They also tend to have more negative reactions to sexual abuse when their relationship with the abuser is close. An experience with a stranger appears to be less damaging and less disturbing than one with someone in their own family. Children in such situations feel there has been a violation of the trust and respect due between those who are close. When the two features are combined, wide age difference and intimacy within the family, the most negative experiences occur.

'I was disgusted that someone as old as that, more than thirty, should expose himself to me in the park. I was only ten at the time and I felt he was very old' (female student, 19 years).

'When my own father started getting sexy with me when I was about eleven I got all confused and ashamed. He must have been about forty. I was well developed and he kept touching my breasts. I was so shocked I had trouble going out with men in my later years' (female student, 38 years).

OTHER FACTORS EVIDENT IN CHILD SEXUAL ABUSE

Girls in the country in Australia are more likely to be sexually abused than girls in urban areas. These are children who live on farms or in rural communities with less than 5000 population or whose fathers' occupations are classed as agricultural. Finkelhor's American study also found this to be so.

And in Australia girls of low-income families tend to be the sexual victims of older partners somewhat more than those in higher-income families. Mothers who have a low level of education tend to have daughters who may be sexually abused. But overall, when measures of income, education and occupational status are assessed, child sexual abuse is prevalent at all levels of society, although in the lower-income families it still appears more likely.

Particularly vulnerable to child sexual abuse are girls who have lived for periods of their childhood without a father because of death, separation or divorce. This is not surprising, since in many ways such girls are not only unprotected but new male partners of the mother, a stepfather together with stepbrothers perhaps, may come to live in the same house. Girls often report that friends of stepfathers in particular, who visit see an opportunity for sexual experience with a girl child of the family.

While the use of alcohol by abusers is not established as an accompanying factor, the excessive use of alcohol in a family, marital unhappiness, and mother's inadequacies due to illness may be significant factors in a daughter being abused.

No clear evidence is forthcoming that any single family factor is common to children who are sexually abused. Some generations ago it was assumed that geographically isolated families of low income where a child had inadequate parents were the most likely setting for child sexual abuse. Rather the evidence shows that there are more complex causes, among which such family problems may play a part.

Nor does the evidence show any increase in our society of child sexual abuse, simply because there are few comparative studies from previous generations to compare with the results of current investigations. The idea that child sexual abuse is on the increase may be due more to an increased awareness of the problem and greater publicity given by the media to such matters. The impression is conveyed, perhaps erroneously, that child sexual abuse is on the increase.

The evidence may indeed indicate the contrary, since in Western societies children are now more protected than during the Industrial Revolution. Because they spend more of their childhood in schools rather than the work place and are legally more secure and are sheltered by care givers, the opportunities for child sexual abuse appear to be less.

SOME TYPICAL CASES OF CHILD SEXUAL ABUSE

The ten cases from our Australian study cited in abbreviated form below are examples of children who have had experiences

173

either with a stranger or with someone known to them. They do not include those sexually abused by close members of their own families. These latter are dealt with in our next chapter on 'Children with Relatives'.

Case 1:   girl aged 5. Male friend of the family about 40 years of age baby-sat, and while tucking her up in bed caressed her sexually. Girl too scared to tell parents.

Case 2:   boy aged 8. Genitals fondled by stranger in public lavatory. Offender (about 20) offered sweets. Boy told friend but no one else.

Case 3:   girl aged 9. Male friend of family, thought to be about 45 years of age, fondled her in a sexual way and persuaded her to let him touch her sexual organs. Girl told no one.

Case 4:   girl aged 9. Male friend of sister, aged about 17 years, touched her sex organs in lounge while waiting to take sister on a date, several times. Girl told no one.

Case 5:   boy aged 12. Strange man about 20 years old masturbated in front of boy in public park, threatened violence if he ran away. Boy told father.

Case 6:   girl aged 10. With older female friend of 18 engaged in mutual sexual fondling and exploration. Girl told no one.

Case 7:   girl aged 8. Male cousin aged 16 years forced her into intercourse by threatening to beat her. In painful distress, girl told sister, who told mother. Cousin banned from the house.

Case 8:   girl aged 11. Male friend of family called 'uncle', aged about 38 years, attempted intercourse with her at his home. Girl told no one but refused to visit him again.

Case 9:   boy aged 13. With female cousin aged 20 engaged in kissing, flirting and fondling his penis to ejaculation, every week for six months. Told no one.

Case 10:   girl aged 13. Stranger about 25 years old exhibited his genitals on way home from school. Girl told mother who informed police, but no one was identified.

It will be noticed that few of these occurrences were reported to anyone except a friend. Fewer than 5% of the experiences described by the students in this survey were reported to adults and only 2% were brought to the attention of authorities. Most children carry the memories of these experiences without sharing their anxieties with anyone. Indeed, many of them reported that our survey was the first opportunity they had had of mentioning their experiences to anyone.

SOME INTERNATIONAL COMPARISONS

Our findings regarding the prevalence of child sexual abuse and other features of the problem are not dissimilar to those reported in other countries. Comparisons are difficult to make however, because different studies draw upon different samples of the population such as the age groups assessed, they use different methods of research and may even have different definitions of what constitutes child sexual abuse.

It is generally agreed that the size of the problem is usually underestimated because of various factors. If clinical or criminal samples are taken, we know that these represent a very small percentage of cases, since the vast majority of cases go unreported. Only the more serious offences, that is, more serious in legal terms, are brought to the attention of the authorities such as a medical centre or the police, and even then not all of these involve official action. General surveys of the population have been done in the USA and Britain but because of the nature of the topic subjects may be inhibited from giving full and frank answers. Samples of student populations are also subject to bias, as are all studies which ask for recollections from adults of events occurring in childhood. [3]

Nevertheless there is general support for the view that the problem of child sexual abuse is widespread, and is especially harmful for girls. A survey of San Francisco women found 28% of them to have been sexually abused before the age of 14 years, a figure similar to our Australian study. An American survey of women students gives a figure of 22% and a Canadian study gives 19%, although this last study only included women who as girls had been threatened to force them to participate. A Swedish study in 1983 gives a figure as low as 9% of women and a British survey reports 12% of females. Low though these figures are in comparison with our own estimates, the actual numbers are still large. From his British study Dr Tony Baker estimates that there are 4 500 000 adults in Britain who were sexually abused as children. He also suggests that over one million British children will be molested before the age of 15 years.

Figures for boys are difficult to gather since it is only recently that boys were thought of as victims. Some surveys show that compared with our 9% of Australian boys, American boys number 9%, British 8% and Swedish 3%. For boys and girls alike, studies in all countries show child sexual abuse to be prevalent at all social levels.

There is also widespread evidence to show that the years between 8 and 11 are the most dangerous sexually for children, as our Australian study suggests. This is shown in American, Canadian and British research, as is the fact that the majority of perpetrators of child sexual abuse are male, not elderly, and are known to the children victimised. All studies report a sizeable incidence of child sexual abuse within families. In addition all studies also report the negative and continuing effects of child sexual abuse upon the victims, especially females, who in later life may find such negativisms inhibiting a normal happy adult sex life, even though only about 5% of cases described involved child sexual intercourse. Some studies specifically assessing the effects of child sexual abuse consistently report low self-esteem on the part of victims.

WHY CHILDREN NEED TO KNOW ABOUT CHILD SEXUAL ABUSE

Research has shown that those who are sexually ignorant are most prone to sexual difficulties. Ignorant young children produce misleading myths which may prevent sound understanding well into married life. Ignorant adolescents are more likely to produce teenage pregnancies, which often have difficult consequences for themselves and their families. And ignorant adults are more prone to sexual mishaps such as clumsy love-making, sexual tensions and venereal disease. Knowledge, while not an infallible solution, is the key to most situations children face, not least the danger of sexual abuse.

Because of the prevalence of child sexual abuse for a sizeable section of our child population it is obvious to us, as to most professionals and child care givers, that children should be warned to resist the sexual blandishments and suggestions of adults. Many parents hesitate to do this and many programs of sex education do not include such items, simply because of the misguided notion that a child's sexual innocence should not be disturbed. Such a view is self-contradictory, since a child will certainly be more disturbed by an experience of being molested sexually than by anything parents or teachers will tell them.

Such hesitation is also based upon the mistaken notion that it may destroy the trust children have for adults. But what is more destructive of such trust than a sexual incident in which children may be persuaded against their will, bullied or threatened into an activity which they feel to be wrong, and made to feel so guilty that they are ashamed to tell anyone?

One of the most basic needs of children, if they are to be protected from sexual abuse, is to know about sexuality, which includes being aware of their own sexual organs. General warnings may only leave children bewildered and confused if they have no clues as to what adults may be warning them about. So information from parents about sexuality from the early years, and a sequential sex education in primary schools, both provide a context in which protective education can be effective. The fact that those aged between 8 and 11 are most at risk is a compelling argument for sex education in the primary (or elementary) school years, since children can acquire from a very early age a general knowledge about their own sexuality which helps to protect them against its violation.

But with or without effective sex education programs, children need to be helped more specifically on how to deal with sexually threatening situations involving adults. Fortunately we do not need to start from zero in these matters, since many programs have been devised in various countries for parents and teachers. The basic principles of such programs are very similar and have proved effective whether taught informally at home or in a more structured way in a school setting as part of the curriculum. These basic principles involve the simple directions of 'No', 'Go' and 'Tell'.[4]

Say 'No'

Children should be taught their right to say 'No' to adults if asked to do anything they feel to be wrong. They need to be taught the difference between good and bad touching, and that they have the right to reject touching or caressing which they don't like. It is better initially to emphasise what they like or dislike rather than right or wrong, since young children have very limited moral perceptions. Their right to say 'No', should be made clear, and apply not only to strangers but to people they know, including members of their own family. No one, including those nearest and dearest to them, has the right to touch children in certain ways if they object. Saying 'No' will also come easier if children are told that there are certain parts of the body most people regard as private. It helps, of course, if parents or teachers can talk about the sex organs without being coy or embarrassed and can use the correct names, not merely the general phrase 'private parts'.

Saying 'No' also involves refusing bribes of sweets, money or other rewards, and especially resistance to threats of force or the use of blackmail. Because these threats may be frightening to children, the next step is also essential.

Go

Children need to feel safe and they should be taught to remove themselves as quickly as possible from any person who makes them feel uncomfortable or threatened. Emphasis can be put upon feeling safe, staying safe and seeking safety if in any way a child feels a dangerous situation has occurred. Children need to be taught to seek safety and remove themselves if they so wish, no matter what an adult may say or do. Admittedly it may be difficult to teach children who are naturally trusting to identify what are dangerous situations for them and who are dangerous people. But once they perceive danger it is best to go. For this reason, the availability of 'safety houses' in a neighbourhood around schools may be part of the program, providing a haven for a child threatened by stranger danger. But children also need to be taught how to be safe if worried by someone they know, even their own family members.

Tell

This is not only important for the child concerned, to unburden fears and ensure they feel safe once removed from potential threat. It is also important from the point of view of other children who may be further victims if the sexual abuser is allowed to continue unchecked.

Teaching children to tell is a basic skill they need for all kinds of emergency – feeling ill, witnessing an accident, calling an ambulance or the fire brigade – as well as more personal dangers such as the activities of a child sexual abuser. Since the vast majority of child sexual abuse incidents go unreported, it seems a fundamental principle to encourage children to tell someone they can trust. The problem is, whom? Case studies indicate, and we have cited some examples in this chapter, that parents who are told about a friend who is a molester may be totally disbelieving of their child and may even punish a child for being a liar. Our survey shows that many children expect to be disbelieved by their parents or feel they might be punished if they report sexual matters. Even so, it is vital that children be taught to tell someone, even if disbelieved the first time, and to go on telling someone else until they are believed.

There are books, videos and films available based upon the 'No', 'Go' and 'Tell' principles, mostly derived from America where such programs have operated for several years. Australian and other readers will find some relevant references to these materials in Freda Briggs' valuable book.[4]

12
CHILDREN WITH RELATIVES: INCEST

Case 1: boy cousin aged 9 staying the night with girl aged 10. He exhibited genitals to her, tried to touch her genitals, but she refused.

Case 2: uncle aged about 38 caressed girl aged 11 when looking after her for the day. Girl sworn to secrecy, told no one. Activity repeated over several months.

Case3: father with daughter began intercourse when daughter aged 7. Continued for five years, until younger daughter replaced her. Mother told but refused to believe. Mother ill, father alcoholic.

These cases illustrate the wide range of sexual experiences children report as having occurred with relatives. By relatives we include more distant relations such as uncles and aunts, cousins, and nieces and nephews, and closer relationships in the nuclear family such as siblings and parents. Also included are step-parents and step-siblings where a re-marriage has occurred after a divorce, resulting in what is now called a blended family.

We have already seen that the family provides many opportunities for sexual education through observing normal intimate day-to-day activities such as the bathing, abluting, dressing and undressing of its members. The wider network of relatives, as well as the more closely knit group of close relatives, also provides opportunities for more overt sexual activities.

To avoid sensationalising the evidence it should be noted that more than 65% of the students in our Australian survey reported no such incidents during their childhood. Of the 35% who did report such incidents, about two-thirds described experiences they had had as children under the age of 12 with child relatives, principally with cousins and siblings. Much of this, as we have reported in Chapter 10, is similar to experience with other non-related children, namely a natural exploration of sex organs and an expression of normal curiosity.

A WORKING DEFINITION OF INCEST

The word 'incest' is commonly thought of as covering all sexual acts between blood relatives, and many readers may tend to label all the cases we have cited as examples of incest. This, however, would be a mistake, since there are two ways of defining incest. The legal definition, which specifies incest as a crime, covers the act of sexual intercourse between persons closely related by blood. Laws may differ from country to country and from state to state about the closeness of the blood relationship included. But according to this legal definition, less than one per cent of the experiences described in our study can be called incest.

However, there is a psychological definition which we prefer to use for 'incestuous' experiences, namely those sexual experiences which cover a wide range from the exhibiting and touching of sexual organs through to the full sexual act, not only by blood relatives but by all relatives within a family where there is a psychologically dependent relationship. This may then include step-parents and half-brothers and -sisters, and covers the growing number of blended families in our society. On this broader definition some few cases can be identified as legal incest, but the majority can be more accurately defined as 'incestuous relationships' or 'intra-family sexual experiences'. This is not to minimise the seriousness, for children especially, of many of these happenings, but it does provide a broader perspective.

HOW PREVALENT ARE INTRA-FAMILY SEXUAL EXPERIENCES?

We have distinguished events which occur between children related to each other, often an experience caused by natural sexual curiosity, from those which occur between more closely related individuals involving what may be termed child sexual abuse by a relative who is much older than the child concerned. These latter cases involve adult relatives who exploit their close relationship, and their power and authority, to persuade children to provide them with some kind of sexual experience.

Consequently we now report on two categories of intra-family sexual experiences which may cause the greatest concern, those involving sibling with sibling and those involving a child with an adult relative.

Sibling with sibling

In describing their experiences with other children before the age of 12, about 11% of the students indicate they had had such a sexual experience with a sibling between the ages of 8 and 12. This was about the same percentage as had had sexual experiences with cousins. The Finkelhor (USA) study we have already cited estimates 13% for both categories, mostly in the years 8 to 11. Most were with a sibling over 8 years of age and most were heterosexual in nature. In our Australian study the vast majority of the experiences with siblings were heterosexual explorations of the sex organs, the same sex games played with friends and distant relatives such as cousins.

However, when reviewing sibling experiences from the ages of 13 to 16 years we must remember that for most teenagers this would be during their post-pubertal time of development. These mainly brother–sister sexual activities at this age may be mutually desired experiences. On the other hand they could be more in the nature of exploitation on the part of an older sibling with a younger teenager. As such they resemble child or adolescent sexual abuse more than the childish sexual exploration of equals.

Typical of this kind of exploitation experience are

Case 4: girl aged 17 and brother aged 14. Heavy petting over two years almost to intercourse, terminated when mother found out.

Case 5: boy aged 18 with sister aged 13. Fondling and exploration of sex organs and attempted sexual inter-course, which terminated the activity.

During this post-pubertal age the sexual drive may be quite strong and difficult for teenagers to control, unless they are counselled wisely by parents. Where both parents are at work there are plenty of opportunities in the home for siblings to seek sexual experiences, especially after school or during school holidays. The evidence indicates boys to be somewhat more frequently the initiators of sibling with sibling sexual activity in the teenage years.

Children with adult relatives

Using the measure of age differences between a child and the other person, and applying it to adult relatives, we find the following experiences described. It will be seen that girls in practically all these experiences are at greater risk than boys.

In our sample, 18 girls had had experiences with a father or a stepfather. Three of these involved sexual intercourse but the majority were experiences of sexual fondling and mutual masturbation with the daughter. Nearly all the experiences described occurred several times, often over months or years. One distressed girl reported sexual fondling by her father when she was aged 7, 9 and 11 years and so she became frightened to be left alone with him. Another reports her father gradually increasing his sexual activities from kissing and hugging sexually when she was 13, to genital fondling when she was 14, and almost sexual intercourse when she was 15. Only one boy reports sexual abuse by his father, an attempt to get him to engage in mutual masturbation.

Another 8 girls reported sexual experiences with grandfathers. One at 5 years old was subjected to a grandfather revealing his genitals once, an event which left her puzzled for a long time. Another at 7 years experienced fondling and sexual touching which caused her grandfather to ejaculate, which made her very frightened of him from that time. With one exception all the grandfather experiences occurred before the child was 9 years. No boys reported such experiences.

One girl recalls sexual fondling by her mother when she was 15 years and her mother was in her late forties. And one boy remembers genital stroking and fondling by his mother when he was about 8 years old which went on at bathtime for several months. As we have noted this low incidence is probably due to the intimate bond between a mother and child which tends to inhibit sexual activities by mothers.

A further 21 girls had had experiences with uncles, which does not include 'honorary' uncles who are usually close friends of father's, given the title of uncle. These honorary uncles are much more numerous as child sex abusers, using their closeness with the family to make overtures to the children. Most legal uncles seem to choose girls between 9 and 11 years, mainly pubertal. The three boys in our study who described uncle activities were 12 to 14 years. Among the girls, there was only one case of intercourse by an uncle although there were several described as attempted intercourse. The majority of cases were exhibiting or fondling of sex organs.

In contrast, six boys and no girls report experiences with aunts. Practically all cases were post-pubertal boys aged 13 to 16 years seduced by an older woman using the occasion of a solitary visit by a nephew.

One unfortunate girl reported that she was sexually abused at 12 by her father touching her sex organs, and again at 16 by a grandfather and an uncle similarly trying to fondle her. She told her mother but was disbelieved.

If the legal definition is taken, then five cases altogether can be seen as legal incest in this sample of Australian students, which represents one half of one per cent of the sample. However, four of these cases are girls, out of 603 this represents about 0.7 of one per cent. Although this seems a small proportion, in Australia's population of just over 16 million people, about half being women, this would lead to an estimate of about 57 000 women who have had sexual intercourse as children or teenagers with an adult blood relative. These figures are disturbingly large.

But taking the psychological definition, thus including all kinds of sexual activities with adult blood relatives, the estimates from our student figures, if typical, would indicate that about 8% of the female population experiences an incestuous relationship. In Australia then, about 650 000 females will have experienced some kind of sexual occurrence in childhood with an adult relative.

Where legal incest is involved, only a small percentage of cases are reported to officials and not all of these result in prosecutions. Similarly, the vast majority of intra-family sexual experiences during childhood with adult relatives are never reported, as our and other studies show. One result of the tendency not to report means that child abusers are free to continue molesting children, most of them within the family, since few are checked from further activities with other children by the law, or even by the pressure of others within a family.

The evidence is also available from our and other related studies that the closer the relationship and the wider the age discrepancy between child and molesting adult, the more traumatic the experience is. Consequently incest and incestuous relationships between children and adults are the most disturbing, frightening and destructive of healthy sexual development of all childhood sexual experiences. Why this is so we explore in a later section. The evidence also shows that girls, who are by far the most numerous victims, show the greatest trauma and negative effects.

Accompanying social factors

As we have noted in cases of children's experiences with adults (Chapter 11), child sexual abuse appears to be related to or accompanied by some verifiable social factors. This is true also of cases of both legal incest and incestuous relationships.

Our study confirms the findings of other research, for example, that rural girls (in other words, those living on farms or in small communities with a population of less than five thousand) are more likely to be the victim of incest or similar intra-family sex than urban girls.

Low-income families, a mother less educated and the presence of inadequate parents because of illness or alcohol seem also to be accompanying social factors in incestuous activities, especially in father–daughter relationships. Unhappy marriages of parents also seem to be relevant.

While we cannot identify these as causes – the connections are far more complex than that – it is clear that inadequate parents and a fragile marriage, of which mother's illness and father's drunkenness may be symptoms, are all factors which make a daughter a possible sexual target.

Why incestuous relationships are destructive

From the evidence of traumatic effects gained from various researches in Australia and America, and from child development studies generally, we can piece together the destructive nature of incestuous relationships. Various groups claim that sexuality practised within the family is beneficial. One of these promotes the slogan 'Sex by year eight before it's too late'.[1]

On the contrary, incest provides a disturbance, whether in traumatic circumstances or not, which impedes, distorts or displaces normal sexual development. We shall illustrate this taking three examples of girls at the pre-pubertal, trans-pubertal and post-pubertal period of development.

Pre-pubertal

Consider a 7-year-old girl and what she thinks about sex, especially about the sexuality of members of her own close family. Family taboos will have discouraged sexual perceptions. To her the family is a close nurturing economic unit. Father is normally seen as provider, bestower of treats and special presents, as grandfathers and uncles are. Any babies born into her family are the result of manufactured activity in the hospitals implanted in mother's stomach by doctors. No sexual activity between father and mother is perceived, or that of any other family relatives. Nakedness is not encouraged after about 5 years of age and showing the sex organs is regarded as naughty and dangerous. If practised it will lead to reprimand and punishment. A girl at this stage is beginning to develop an aversion to boys, although some 'naughty' games may occur with one of them, in satisfying curiosity about the male sex organ.

Suddenly a grown-up member of the family – a father, uncle, grandfather or much older brother – violates these accepted notions the 7-year-old girl has. A male sex organ is perhaps displayed, and areas of her body fondled. Such newly experienced intimacy may be flattering or even pleasurable but it will undoubtedly be puzzling. The adult family member, especially father, is a symbol of authority and trustworthiness, and here he is making unusual and furtive demands which break the rules imposed in modesty training, invoking a feeling of uneasiness or guilt in the child. If, as in most cases, the experience is transitory and not physically painful, the effects may not be traumatic. If force is used and intercourse occurs or is attempted it will be frightening and painful. But it will certainly result in confusion about family roles, poor impulse control by the child, some guilt in relation to mother and perhaps a sexual precociousness not always socially approved. This is not a healthy introduction to sexuality but a distorted, contradictory, uncomfortable and distressing experience.

Trans-pubertal

If we consider a typical 11-year-old girl it is probable we shall see one whose pubertal development has been occurring for almost two years but who has not yet had her first menstruation. She will know that babies result from something her mother and father do together and that marriage is partly a sexual union. However, taboos will operate to limit her perception. Grown-up members of the family, especially the father, are seen as protectors. If her father's endearments or those of any other male members of the family are expressed too strongly, she may be embarrassed and will be vaguely aware of their sexual meaning. If the endearments go too far, then she will become very uncomfortable and try to evade the situation.

Sexual intercourse, exhibiting the sex organs or similar activities she will recognise as a taboo activity for her age group. Although perhaps exciting it will also be a repelling and dangerous activity. Romantic or sexual feelings are to be reserved for a special person when she gets older, and this is perceived as a different kind of feeling to the feeling she has for a father, an elder brother, a grandfather or uncle. An incestuous experience at this stage will most certainly be traumatic, as many cases in our study illustrate. Any excitement experienced will generate guilt and also an enormous sense of betrayal (of the mother especially, if the perpetrator is father) since she will be aware that something is happening that distorts normal family relationships.

It may well be the first time she has seen the sex organs of a fully grown man or received a sexual suggestion of any kind, and this from a man close to her whom she has learned to trust. Sex role confusion will certainly occur and family jealousies and rivalries may result, especially between mother and daughter, and between the daughter and other siblings. Distaste for sexual activities may well occur in the future, leading to a distrust of the other sex at a time when she is beginning to over-come her aversion to them and find a heterosexual friendship possible. Or the opposite could happen, an excessive and early sexual drive in the pursuit of a love which is not a betrayal of trust.

Post-pubertal

Considering a 14-year-old girl, we see a girl with full sexual awareness who is fully developed physically and capable of reproduction. She will know intercourse may lead to pregnancy but will have little knowledge of birth control methods. And she will be aware of possible consequences of family disruption or disharmony if any incestuous relationship is discovered. The closer the relationship, especially if it is with father, the more disturbing the experience will be. If she tells, the providing father may be removed, the family as known will disintegrate and the daughter will be left with the feeling she is responsible for such a disaster.

As an adolescent girl she will need parental support, from her mother as an emotional care giver and father as adviser, sympathiser and sex role model of the male she will eventually hope to marry. If a father–daughter sexual relationship is experienced these models will be denied her, and the normal sexual transition from family to heterosexual friendships may be considerably delayed or clouded with suspicion. Grand-fathers or uncles do not have quite the same effect, but they will destroy a trusting relationship if a sexual encounter occurs, with negative feelings as a result. She will be aware that if she tells her mother, all kinds of unpleasant rows may occur. If the relative is high in family esteem the daughter may be totally disbelieved, as many cases indicate. Either way, suspicions are created about the motives and behaviour of the other sex gener-ally. This is most unfortunate at a time when heterosexual friendships with her male peers should be developing.

Hence we can see that at all stages of development outright incest or incestuous relationships with an adult affect the grow-ing child and adolescent girl negatively. It is a gross distortion to claim it has beneficial and positive effects.

SEDUCTION THEORY AND BLAMING THE VICTIM

The readiness of many adults to disbelieve children's accusations of incest or child sexual abuse by an adult is partly the result of a long tradition of blaming the victim. In this, Sigmund Freud's theory contributed to a misunderstanding of the true situation which has resulted in great unhappiness for countless patients who undertook psychoanalysis. Unfor-tunately many of the assumptions behind Freud's ideas have become part of a popular fallacy, which needs to be discredited.

In his seduction theory, Freud first advanced the view from a number of his women patients' accounts of their childhood that they had been seduced by a male member of their own family, in many cases by the father. From this he deduced that sexual trauma was at the root of many later adult neuroses. But it has been suggested that because incest was regarded as not only unacceptable but unthinkable to his colleagues Freud changed his views and relegated these incest accounts to the realm of fantasy.[2] This helped him develop his well-known Oedipus complex, regarded as a cornerstone of Freudian theory, in which children allegedly dream of sexual union with a parent.

In denying that the incest accounts of his patients were based upon reality, Freud removed the shocking possibilities of a father doing such a thing to his daughter. Instead such actions were relegated to the fantasy life of the child who herself yearns for the incestuous relationship she states as fact. This neatly put the blame on the victim, not the father, as the seducer. A similar strategy of blaming the victim is still to be seen in cases of rape where women are blamed for wearing provocative clothes or make-up, or are said to have encouraged sex by walking alone at night.

So a serious and objective examination of child–adult incest was probably prevented for over seventy years by Freud's change of mind. His denial placed the blame, if incest occurred at all, upon the precocious and provocative sexual wishes of the child. This also laid the foundation for disbelieving children, the dismissal of their accounts as wicked fantasies which were intended to besmirch so-called perfectly respectable adult members of the family.

The evidence we now have, as our figures indicate, is that legal incest and incestuous experiences of children are sufficiently numerous to merit the serious attention of society. They can no longer be dismissed as fantasy (as some therapists amazingly still maintain) but are part of our concern for children to develop sexually in a healthy manner. Incest is certainly not one of those experiences. Where it does occur, children should be comforted and protected, not rejected and blamed or dubbed malicious liars.[3]

But the reactions of adults to the whole question of incest are more complex. Anthropologists have pointed out that practically all cultures condemn incest as a taboo activity. The popular view is that incest is universally regarded as unnatural and inherently repugnant. Yet the opposite view may be advanced, that incest taboos exist as a practical defence against a very natural occurrence which may happen in a family with intimate daily physical contacts. This view seems the most plausible since the incidence of incest is much greater than previously assumed, especially if we use the broader term of 'incestuous relationships', that is intra-family sexual experiences. This view is also more consistent with the reactions of parents to nakedness and other lapses in modesty on the part of children. The fear is that by such behaviour sexual drives or impulses may get out of control.

There is, in addition, the vague distinction between loving sensuality between parent and child and what we have described as abusive and exploitative sexuality. The differences between loving and affectionate support and lustful gestures is surprisingly subtle. It is the parent's responsibility to set limits and control sexual impulses, not the child's.

An illustration of this difficult distinction is made by an American researcher. When children are ill or awaken frightened at night, they are sometimes allowed in the parental bed as a comfort. Often it may be the occasional Sunday morning ritual snuggle together. But when does sharing a bed with a parent pass the limit of sensual enjoyment into a sexual experience, however confusedly it occurs? Clearly these limits must be understood by parents and firmly but lovingly imposed.[4]

WHAT CAN BE DONE ABOUT INTRA-FAMILY SEXUAL RELATIONSHIPS INVOLVING CHILDREN?

We shall answer this question in terms of the two types of incestuous relationships we defined earlier; sibling with sibling, and child with adult experiences within the family.

Sibling with sibling sexual experiences which may be brother and sister, sister with sister, or brother with brother where the children are of roughly the same age, may be simply sexual explorations arising from natural curiosity mainly about the sex organs. As such they can be disregarded or accepted as normal, similar to the experiences children have with other children who are friends. Sister with sister, and brother with brother, are more likely to be in the sex game exploration category.

But brother–sister experiences may become established, not merely a once or twice occurrence, and lead to an unhealthy sexual attachment, which can only result in the long run in difficult if not disastrous consequences. It is important for parents to be able to recognise the signals which generally occur when brother–sister experiences become sexually intense. They may behave like a courting couple, demonstrating affection to each other more than normally, such as holding hands or hugging each other. The converse may occur when a child shows anxieties at being left alone with a brother or sister. Or siblings may betray signs of discomfort or confusion if a parent finds them alone together unexpectedly.

It is important to remain calm, and in talking with the siblings to help them disclose what really happened. Suspicions may be without any foundation but it is better to try to bring such matters out into the open than to let the suspicion continue. Often a sympathetic discussion will prevent any further activity, but more drastic action such as the rearrangement of sleeping quarters may be necessary where a younger child is being exploited by an older brother or sister. Obviously the older one may need more attention and counselling, as the possible initiator.

There are many more problems when adult members of the family sexually abuse a child. More distant relatives such as uncles and aunts are, we know from the evidence, among such abusers. In terms of helping a child cope with such an occurrence general references can be made in 'No, Go, Tell' programs, but once an event has occurred there are several guidelines which may be followed. First it is vital to be approachable and to listen sympathetically to what a child has to say, no matter how respectable the adult who is named may be. Again, it is important to remain calm and particularly not to assume that a child is guilty of malicious make-believe, a reaction of far too many parents. A child will usually be more in need of comfort and reassurance, even before he or she is willing to relate any such experience. The more unpleasant and frightening the experience has been, the more the child will be in need of comfort and have difficulties in talking about it.

Once it has been established that a child has had a frightening or distasteful experience it is vital that steps be taken to prevent a recurrence. Embarrassing though it may be, adult offenders must be talked to and some plain speaking is required, however close the relationship within the family. Most sexual activities of this kind are criminal offences. Not only must the child immediately concerned be protected, but other potential child victims also. There is a natural reluctance to report these matters to the authorities, because of the disgrace it may cause the family, yet it is far better than allowing the misdemeanours to continue.

Our major concern in this book is with children as victims or potential victims. But it is important to point out that the vast majority of child molestors are not sexual monsters, but inadequate, frustrated and rather pathetic men who cannot gain satisfaction in an adult sexual relationship. The evidence is that if remedial services were provided by society such men would welcome help. Community services of this kind are as yet comparatively undeveloped but are needed much more than long prison sentences.

Father–daughter incestuous relationships, which may include legal incest, are much more difficult and intimidating to a family than events involving uncles or grandfathers. Professional help is certainly needed in such cases. In addition to listening and giving comfort adults must protect the child; this is vital. Many mothers are reluctant to take any action because to remove a father may take away the economic basis of the family. But far too often a child is removed into a children's institution, when it is she who needs the support and care of her mother in the security of her own home. It is wise in most cases for the father to remove himself voluntarily from the home, until such time as the child can trust him and he has received adequate counselling.

Since incest concerns families and key members of a family need help, as well as protection, community family programs such as those developed in some parts of the United States are needed. Such work is in California based on self-help family groups, not unlike Alcoholics Anonymous, and high success rates are reported, with little recurrence of sexual offences. Group psychotherapy is needed for young children, and also man–woman counselling teams to deal with sexually abused adolescents.[5]

Outside America, societies are becoming more aware of these

problems. As awareness based upon reliable research increases it is to be hoped that more remedial facilities and preventive programs will be provided. The figures we produce are sufficient, we believe, to merit concerted action and the concern and involvement of all social agencies, with support of adequate legislation.

13
FIRST SEXUAL EXPERIENCES

'My first real date was when I was 13. I was so nervous I could hardly talk to her. We went to the Saturday (movie) matinee and held hands. I sweated so much it wasn't pleasant, all slippery, so awkward I vowed I'd never do it again' (Australian male student, 20 years).
'This boy took me to a dance at school. But he was two inches shorter than me and he couldn't dance. I felt sorry for him, but my satin shoes got trampled on. I was 14' (Australian female student, 22 years).

Dating is often thought of by parents as the most important indicator of a growing interest in sex on the part of their children. The occasion of a first date may be accepted gladly by parents, or it may be viewed with foreboding accompanied by many warnings. The anxiety level of parents and their young may be quite high and the morale of the teenagers concerned relatively low. Dating represents 'a coming out', a demonstration of growing maturity and a mixed indicator for parents. If it comes in their opinion too soon, anxieties may be expressed that their youngsters are too young. If dating is viewed as late, parents may fear their teenager is not normal physically or socially or they may harbour hidden fears of their offspring's homosexuality, especially if he is male.

We shall be treating the subject of homosexuality, a preference for one's own sex whether male or female, later in this chapter. The percentage of practising homosexuals in our society is somewhere between 10% and 20%, depending on how it is defined. For these one in five to one in ten in our population, first heterosexual dating can be a misleading indicator.

There are other first-time sexual experiences, apart from

dating, which are more important indicators for parents and teachers in assessing the sexual maturing of children and teen-agers. Until recently the time when such events as first menstruation, first wet dreams and first intercourse could be expected were a matter for guesswork or guess-timates. But evidence is accumulating that such events, and other sexual experiences, are occurring earlier in children's lives. We have already reviewed the incidence and impact of earlier sexual maturing (see Chapter 1), and the possible reasons for such happenings. We now provide some evidence for when we might expect certain experiences to happen to our children and thus outline a more realistic picture of what is normal sexual development.

WHAT IS NORMAL?

Before we review this evidence we must state that normality covers a very wide range of both age and quality of experience. Early and late developers come within the range of normal, not only those clustered around the average age of the onset of adolescence. It is quite normal to find within a school class of 12-year-olds whose ages are within twelve months of each other those with the bodies of children, of limited height and with few traces of pubertal growth, alongside those who have the well-developed bodies of young adults. It is quite within what we consider normal that some will reveal pubertal changes from 7 or 8 years of age, beginning at that time two or more years of growth in height, weight, chest development and pubertal hair. It is also normal if these changes do not begin until after 12 years of age, this at a time when half of the age group may have almost completed that growth process.

Obviously there are medical conditions which may unduly delay or speed up hormonal growth in children, and medical consultation and appropriate treatment may then be necessary. Such cases are rare and for the vast majority it is best for nature to take its course following the genetic patterns established for each child at conception.

So what is the range of ages at which we can expect certain

sexual experiences to happen to our children and teenagers? And what is the range of experiences which might then occur? Answers to these questions will help us become better care-givers of children and enable us to answer the needs of the young at such times.

Our estimates and descriptions are estimates of ages and experiences based upon students recollecting their develop-ment during the Australian survey and supplemented by what we know from medical records or other surveys in similar countries with a Western industrialised society. Some of the evidence has already been described in earlier chapters, and may be repeated here so that we can gain an overview of current trends. In presenting these first-time experiences we begin with the earliest experiences and proceed through to those experienced at later stages.

FIRST MASTURBATION EXPERIENCES

'Masturbation' is a misleading word because it is used to cover self-touching and exploring the sex organ, self-fondling for comfort, self-fondling for pleasure and self-fondling for both pleasure and ejaculation. This last activity is what most adults recognise as the masturbatory activities of grown-ups, but the term is also used for the activities seen in early childhood.

The evidence appears to show that from 18 months to 2 years young children have mastered the use of hands and fingers sufficiently to explore practically all parts of their bodies. In exploring their sex organ they soon experience a sense of comfort in touching and stroking it, an experience often becoming habitual in the same way as thumb-sucking. This kind of habitual comfort-seeking is often well established from 2 to 4 years of age. As we have already noted, if it is dealt with in too punitive a manner children will react by showing a need of more comfort and increase the activity. They soon learn to do this secretively when no reprimanding adult is about. Because of the fear of punishment, associated guilt is then experienced.

Fondling the sex organ for comfort merges into deliberate

fondling for pleasure. This may be an intermittent activity at any stage from 3 years up to 9 or 10 years, done when the child is in bed or alone, such as when watching television. Thumb-sucking may also accompany this activity, thus increasing the pleasure experienced. Teachers in pre-school and the early primary school years report frequent activities of this kind. Many adults sensibly use gentle dissuasion and train children not to engage in such pleasure-seeking activity in public.

There is little information about when masturbation to ejaculation occurs, since there is a scarcity of research evidence on such matters. It is thought to begin for most boys at about the age of 10. Group masturbation among boys is quite common from the ages of 11 to 15 and older, and this activity most certainly leads to ejaculation as we would expect in the pubertal development years and beyond.

When our Australian students were asked when they first learned to arouse themselves, an indirect way of asking about masturbation, 4% said between the ages of 8 and 10 years, 21% from 11 to 13 years, 51% between 14 and 16 years and 23% from 17 years onwards. It is significant that boys by far out-number girls from 8 to 13 years, and that after this age girls then outnumber boys – that is, the age of first masturbation has a distinct sex difference.

It is generally accepted that boys come to this activity much earlier than girls simply because a boy's sex organ is external and invites earlier and easier manipulation. In contrast a girl's major sex organ is mainly internal and the outer part of the vulva is less accessible and more difficult to manipulate than is a penis for a boy. The existence of a clitoris may not be known by girls until late childhood or even the teenage years. Boys also are more readily aroused to erection by motions of a vehicle or by accidental rubbing of clothes. All this despite the fact that on average girls are earlier developers than boys, that is, the age at which the menarche occurs is lower than that for its male equivalent.

During masturbation for ejaculation or orgasm, erotic fantasies tend to develop, linked with the natural need for a sexual partner. Since such partnerships are still taboo for young teenagers it is a playful form of mental exploration as well as an exercise in relief from sexual tension. Erotic fantasies of males are better documented than females, as we know from various surveys described in the Kinsey and the Hite reports. Here are some more recent descriptions.

'When I was a teenager I used to wank [masturbate] with the picture in my head of a female I'd seen in a magazine, usually a film star. I'd do it every night, sometimes for months at a time' (male student, 18 years).
'At first it gave me great pleasure just to touch myself between the legs. But when I'd been to the beach I'd imagine I was with one of those bronzed handsome life-savers. He'd be doing it to me' (female student, 21 years).

Evidence indicates erotic fantasy during masturbation to be a universal experience among fully developed men and women, even when they are married. It is therefore not surprising that it is an experience known to most teenagers, whose need for a release of erotic fantasy may be greater than that of adults.

FIRST SEXUAL EXPERIENCES WITH OTHER CHILDREN

After sex exploration of one's self the earliest sexual experiences appear to be some kind of genital exploration with another child. As we have seen, this is usually done in twosomes, between those of the same sex or between those of both sexes. Since the greatest taboo is on seeing, touching or fondling the other sex's organ, heterosexual explorations come a little later than same-sex activity.

About 10% of children's sexual experiences with another child occur before the age of 5 years, in simple games of 'Mothers and Fathers', and dressing and undressing. It increases dramatically from 6 to 9 years when 43% of children have experiences of this kind for the first time. Just over 49% report it occurring for the first time between 10 and 12 years, the peak appearing to be the years between 9 and 10.

The older the children the more elaborate and sexually disguised the games played will be. This gives way in teenagers to much more overt erotic play, leading to heavy petting and usually stopping short of intercourse.

Many adults are only vaguely aware that children have sexual experiences with other children and are rather relieved that such happenings are not brought to their attention. However, when children are discovered or adult attention is drawn to such experiences, the reaction is all too often negative and condemnatory.

'We were pretending to be a mother and father [boy and girl playmate aged about 7 years] cuddling each other with our clothes on, when my mother caught us. She sent her [the girl] home immediately, and scolded me about how naughty I'd been. I was left bewildered because I did not know until much later what was bad about it. The girl was not allowed to play with me again' (male student, 19 years).
'Mum told my father when he got home from work, and he gave us the strap. She'd found my brother and me taking our clothes off and looking at our things. I cried a lot and was told it served me right. At 6 years old I was supposed to know better.' (female student, 23 years).

Not all adults react in this negative way. Many parents are aware that most children at some time express their sexual curiosity in various play themes. In other words they recognise it as a normal play activity of the young. Only when it becomes obsessive, involves rough or painful experiences or frightens children, should adults intervene. Even then reassurances and simple explanations of why such things should not happen are better than vague warnings and punishments.

Parents may be less relaxed and accepting of teenagers exploring their sexuality together. Mutual masturbation games may be discovered between teenage boys, or a teenage girl and boy may be found in various activities of intimacy. Both activities are normal in the sense that they are natural expressions of the sexual drive and at some time or other will be experienced by very many teenagers. Again, vague warnings and threats are of little use. Rather than condemnation teenagers should be receiving some education about the place of sexuality in developing human relationships and the importance of love and respect.

Nevertheless, teenage experiences are different from those of children with other children. Many teenagers will have reached adolescence and have the capacity to reproduce, that is to conceive a child. Certain sexual limits need to be brought to their attention, and restraints and courtesies discussed. We shall see more precisely what is involved when we discuss 'first dating'.

FIRST EXPERIENCE OF MENSTRUATION

The first experience of menstruation or first period in girls is often called the menarche, from the Greek meaning 'month' (*men*) and 'beginning' (*arche*). The popular view is that 14 years is the time the menarche can be expected. Many mothers' expectations and even sex education courses seem to be based upon this misconception.

The average age for the menarche, as we know from medical records in many Western industrialised countries, is in the first half of the twelfth year. Among Aboriginal girls in Australia and Maori girls in New Zealand the average is estimated to be nearer the twelfth birthday. But dependence upon averages can be misleading, especially if we are concerned to prepare girls for what is to happen and help them to cope with this first experience adequately. Some 68% of our Australian women students report that they experienced the menarche beween 11 and 13, but some 4% report that it happened at 10 years or before. Only 27% say it occurred between 14 and 16 years, and 1% after 17 years of age. These figures are similar to those shown in surveys in Britain, America and other countries.

The spread or range of when the menarche is normal is very wide, but we should be aware of the fact that it is likely to be earlier rather than later. Parents and teachers can be forewarned of its occurrence by the usual indications of pubertal growth, which begin about two years before the menarche. These include increases in a girl's height and weight, muscular and breast development and the growth of hair under the arms and in the pubic area. Some if not all of these indications of pubertal growth can be determined by any observant adult who is in close contact with girls. Once they are identified, preparing the girl for the event should not be delayed for long if unpleasant and frightening effects are to be avoided. We have already illustrated (in Chapter 7) how alarming the first menstruation can be if a girl is totally unprepared.

Although most girls report distressing experiences because of inadequate preparation, it is useful to note what happens when adults have wisely anticipated the event.

'When I was 10 my mother talked to me about getting periods. She told me why it happens and showed me how to use a sanitary towel. Until that time I didn't know all women have periods, not even my own mother. A year later it happened during the night and I just went to the bathroom and got a towel and told my mother the next day. I was anxious but not scared out of my wits as I knew some of my friends were' (female student, 21 years).

'A teacher at school noticed I was growing fast, my breasts were getting bigger. I think I was about 12. She took me aside and told me about menstruation and I think talked to my mother. So I was all ready when it happened and no hassles' (female student, 19 years).

Perhaps an exception in one case is the girl who was not only prepared but enjoyed a family celebration a few days later.

'My mother and elder sister told me all about it well in advance, told me what to expect. Mum and Dad talked about it openly when it happened, saying it was great to see me growing. We had a party to celebrate the next Saturday. I think it was a great help for my younger sister and brother to hear about it' (female student, 18 years).

This girl added she hoped to do the same for her children when they were growing up – a refreshing approach that needs to be encouraged.

FIRST EXPERIENCE OF A WET DREAM

For boys the nearest equivalent experience to a girl's menstruation is wet dreams, often called nocturnal or night emissions. This is the involuntary ejaculation of semen often during sleep, which signals the full sexual maturing of the male. There is little direct evidence of when this occurs since medical records are not kept of the first time it occurs in a boy's life. On average a boy's development is about nine months later than girls so we might infer that 13 is the average age for a first wet dream.

Our Australian student data reveal a slightly earlier age. About 10% of male students reported their first wet dream to be at age 10 or before, 53% at age 11 to 13, 36% at age 14 to 16, and about 2% at 17 or older. This would indicate the average age to be nearer 12 than 13.

We have already shown how disturbing if not frightening this event can be for boys who have no knowledge beforehand that it is going to occur. There is some anecdotal evidence to indicate that the vast majority of boys are ignorant of what is likely to happen and do not know how to deal with it.

'It happened one night. I don't know exactly when but I may have been in my early teens. There was just a nasty sticky mess on the bed-clothes and on my pyjamas. I got into a panic and tried to wash the sheets and my 'jama trousers in the bathroom when no one was about. I thought I had a disease or something' (male student, 24 years).
'The first time it happened my mother cleaned up the sheets. Nothing was said and I was very anxious. Then Dad talked to me and told me to control myself. No explanation, just it seemed I was some kind of pervert' (male student, 19 years).

Some boys report that nothing was said and the silence was difficult to handle. But many did not elaborate on the experience, reporting only the age at which it first occurred. It is, like the subject of masturbation, a topic most people avoid. For many it is an anxiety-generating beginning to the more voluntary experience of masturbating to ejaculation.

Boys can be prepared in advance and their anxieties relieved, as with girls and their first menstruation. They should be told that it happens to practically all boys as they are growing up, that it means full sexual maturity has begun and this indicates that conception of a baby is possible. Such explanations will also provide an opportunity to talk about teenage sexuality, the responsibility of boys in sexual relationships and other related matters.

Signals for adults to prepare boys are, as in girls approaching the menarche, the normal appearance of pubertal growth. These include increase in height and weight, muscular and chest development and the growth of facial hair, and hair in the armpits, in the pubic region and elsewhere. The breaking of a boy's voice tends to come a little later in physical development.

The conspiracy of silence about wet dreams is very wide-spread and probably causes boys as much continued anxiety and guilt as menstruation does in girls. Parents in particular should be alert to help a boy over this difficult experience, although not all boys have to deal with wet dreams. They may, however, experience unwelcome erections, and ejaculation may occur when they don't expect it. [1]

FIRST HETEROSEXUAL DATING

It is not surprising to see that early sexual maturing, as indicated by the average age of first menstruation in girls and of first wet dreams in boys, leads to an earlier interest in heterosexual friendships. The outcome of this in most cases is a boy and a girl going out together, an occasion for which the Americanism 'dating' is used.

Heterosexual dating in twosomes is often preceded by boys and girls going around in larger groups, providing a wider social scene in which pairing off occurs. This may be in a school or a social or youth club. Some twosomes, however, may simply arise from chance meetings. The evidence shows that most people go on their first date during their teenage years.

Only one in a hundred of our Australian students reported having their first date before the age of 11. These appear to be very early developers. Some 22% reported that their first date occurred when they were between 11 and 13 years, and 62% when they were between 14 and 16. The average age is 14 years, and up to that age boys report earlier activity than girls.

There is obviously a time lag between the beginnings of adolescence and the first dating, since it takes confidence to go out with a member of the other sex for the first time. Teenagers, especially boys, have to survive the critical and often crude comments of their male peers. They also have to feel confident enough to break away from their previous phase of homosexual or homophilic friendships. Both breaking away from these long-lasting friendships and moving towards a heterosexual friendship can generate great anxieties. Most teenagers, as did those whom we quote at the beginning of this chapter, report it as quite a nerve-wracking and emotionally exhausting business.

First dating usually occurs at a most demanding period of development when body changes are still happening, when new drives and emotions are being experienced for the first time, and when a new set of social and sexual rules have to be learned. The other sex has been for many years only vaguely known, both sexes preferring their own sex from about seven years of age until their teenage years. And teenagers are relatively inexperienced and immature in the exercise of social skills.

At this stage teenagers need support from adults and to be taught these social skills, including the etiquette of a sexual relationship. Yet what girls usually receive are dire warnings of 'going too far' without it being defined what 'too far' is, while boys tend to be warned 'not to get a girl into trouble', again 'the trouble' being only vaguely defined.

Students revealed that what they most appreciated was frank and honest talk from a parent or a trusted adult about the limits to sexual activity they should observe. They are impatient of coy, imprecise and too generalised ideas and want to be told openly about the various levels of sexuality they will encounter. If kissing and hugging are acceptable, what are the limits of fondling? Most teenagers appreciate the distinction of sexual fondling above and below the waist.

But it is not the mechanics of sexual behaviour that is important at this stage so much as talking about human sexuality as an expression of a certain kind of relationship. Sexuality is best saved for those with whom a special closeness is desired, not bestowed on any one. There is evidence to show that young people generally try to behave in this way and do not favour promiscuity.[2] This is of some importance when we look at the earlier age of first intercourse.

FIRST EXPERIENCE OF SEXUAL INTERCOURSE

Many surveys have reported the earlier age at which the young now have their first experience of sexual intercourse. American, British and Swedish researchers have over the last twenty years arrived at this conclusion by direct questioning of young people and by using sources such as medical records. The Swedes in particular have estimated that gradually over the last forty years the average age at first intercourse has dropped from 19 to 16 years.

Our Australian survey indicates a similar trend. Two per cent of all our Australian respondents reported having their first experience by the age of 10 years, 6% between 11 and 13 years and 39% between 14 and 16 years. A further 41% reported having it between 17 and 19 years and the rest after the age of 20. If these figures are accurate, then the middle teens seem to be the average age when first sexual intercourse occurs.

Most adults will find this evidence disturbing for various reasons. It is obvious from the figures that sexual drives are so strong that calls for sexual abstention are frequently not taken seriously. This may be a result of earlier sexual maturing together with a more permissive approach to sexual activity evident in many ways, encouraged by stimulation from the mass media. Perhaps the most disturbing feature of this earlier experience is that less than 25% in Australia indicated that they used contraceptives the first time they had sexual intercourse. This is in contrast to Sweden where a survey from the Swedish Family Planning Association reveals that more than 80% of young people there use some birth control method when first having sexual intercourse.[3]

It is not enough to blame sex education for suggesting to young people that sexual intercourse is acceptable or stimulating them to practise it by 'putting ideas into children's heads'. The evidence is that earlier sexual intercourse is occurring, and has been occurring over many decades in many countries where sex education is non-existent or is taught only to late teenagers. The average age for first intercourse is similar in the USA and New Zealand, where sex education is either not provided or delayed, to the average age in Sweden where sex education begins early.

What sex education in Sweden does is to emphasise quite effectively two matters, which our evaluation of the Swedish syllabus bears out.[4] The first emphasis is on sexual responsibility and their syllabus counsels deferring full sexual activity until old enough to be responsible. But, sensibly, information and advice is given on contraception as part of the education in responsibility. The second emphasis is to make the goal of a sexual relationship one of permanence. This coincides with the concern of the vast majority of young people in Sweden, and in other countries surveyed, to be faithful in a partnership.

So while there is strong evidence for earlier sexual intercourse, there is no evidence for widespread promiscuity. There is every indication that, when given the support and education needed, the young will behave responsibly and that they do in fact seek relationships which will last. Where support and adequate information are not available, then earlier sexual intercourse will still occur, but with much higher rates of teenage pregnancies and other sexual consequences.

HOMOSEXUAL EXPERIENCE IN THE TEENAGE YEARS

Somewhere between one in five and one in ten people have a homosexual experience during their lives. Generally experts suggest that no more than 10% of the adult population are practising homosexuals at any given time. Estimates are difficult to make about the incidence of homosexuality since there are some who are bisexual in practice, engaging in homosexual relationships while still experiencing a permanent heterosexual relationship. We define a homosexual person as one who primarily or solely prefers his/her own sex for a sexual partnership. When men prefer men, the words 'homosexual' or 'gay' are used to describe them. Where women prefer women, the words 'lesbian' or 'gay' are used. As Michael Carrera suggests, 'Homosexuality is not a choice people make, but is a fundamental fact about their personalities.' In other words most homosexuals have little choice about being homosexual, just as most heterosexuals have little choice about being heterosexuals. Although we talk about preference for the same sex, few homosexuals appear to have a choice about such a preference. There are various theories to explain homosexuality but the fact remains that a sizeable proportion in any population will develop into homosexuals and will practise homosexuality. For this reason most sexologists would accept Carrera's views on homosexuality.[5]

Despite this fact and the great amount of writing and publicity about homosexuality, little is known about its early stages in child and adolescent development. During childhood and in the early teenage years children do tend to go through a strong homosexual preference stage, when forming other-sex friendships and heterosexual activities may be strongly resisted. Some prefer to call this phase 'homophilic' rather than homosexual. There is evidence to show that while homosexuals do not make the transition to heterosexuality which the majority makes, they will often hide their same-sex preferences until later. Such are the social pressures that many will engage in heterosexual dating and courtship, and even marry, rather than admit their sexual preference. Indeed, numbers of homosexuals do not recognise themselves as such until later in life, and some then still choose to be 'closet' homosexuals, not willing to come out into the open.

It is therefore very difficult to determine when and how homosexuality begins in any active sense. Consequently in our survey we asked the students if and when after the age of 12 years they first had a sexual experience with someone of the same sex. About 23% of the total group said they had had such an experience, and about 20% were able to identify the age at which they had their first experience. This is almost identical with the one in five frequency we mentioned earlier.

Of those who reported a homosexual experience, 20% said

it occurred when they were between 11 and 13 years, and about 30% say it occurred between the ages of 14 and 16 years. The rest estimated that it occurred after they were 17, or did not specify any age at all. Some of those aged 16 or below may have been reporting homosexual sexual abuse by older partners (see our report in Chapter 11). But since it was mainly males reporting such experiences (and these were only 9% of all males) we are probably identifying a large percentage of genuine mutually agreed homosexual experiences between teenagers of about the same age. Boys report significantly more first homosexual experiences between 11 and 16 years than do girls. Lesbian experiences appear to occur much later.

Parents have often expressed to us their anxiety that a child of theirs will turn out to be homosexual. This may be a negative expression of repulsion at the idea that such a thing could happen in their family, or it may be simply a concern that it will be a source of unhappiness for the child involved, since society still reveals great hostility to homosexuals. Such anxieties are voiced particularly about boys becoming homosexuals and curiously, very rarely about girls becoming lesbians.

It must be said that it is not possible to identify a homosexual child or teenager, or to predict that any youngster will emerge as a homosexual later on. Close same-sex friendships may be a normal homophilic relationship during the childhood and adolescent years. Reluctance to form a heterosexual friendship may be due to natural shyness or slowness in relating to the other sex; it does not necessarily indicate continuing homosexual tendencies. On the other hand there are many who will try heterosexual friendships and to all appearances will be heterosexual, but in reality will gradually become aware that their sexual preferences lie elsewhere.

What can parents do? If young persons begin to understand that they are homosexual, it is to be hoped that they will feel able to talk about it to their parents. Sadly, however, many will feel unable to confide in them since they fear condemnation or rejection. What the young need at such a time and given such a situation is acceptance and support from their own family. It is difficult enough simply to face the fact that one is homosexual, without facing additional difficulties at home. If parents have difficulties accepting homosexuality then they will find it hard to provide the sympathy needed for their son or daughter. Such parents, however, will tend not to know, since their child will not confide in them.

Parents who want to help will provide sympathetic support, for they will know what difficulties lie ahead of their child. They will take the trouble to find out the true facts about homosexuality. They will encourage their child to talk about it and discuss the various ways they can find some social support. Despite their own anxieties and possible feelings of social shame, the best contribution parents can make is an attitude of understanding.[6]

PART THREE
WHAT DOES IT ALL MEAN?

In reviewing the evidence that children are sexual, and by reporting our two major studies, we have demonstrated how ill prepared are children and adolescents to deal with sexuality. Because many of the children's explanations are amusing it is easy to treat them as the natural and rather funny results of immaturity. Children's gaffes and misunderstandings while they are young are a constant source of amusement to adults. This final section deals with the more serious implications of what we have so far presented. The general question 'What does it all mean?' we try to answer at two levels. In Chapter 14 we do so at the practical level, by discussing how to help adults help children. In so doing we review what the long history of sexual deceit does to children and the adult myths about childhood which need to be dispelled. The problem about childhood sexuality is not the children, nor their sexuality; it is the mishandling of it by adults. Consequently we describe what children need from adults in terms of acceptance, sensitivity, honesty and education.

In the final chapter (Chapter 15) we explore some difficult and unresolved issues, beginning with individual and familial differences, the question of morals and values involved in teaching the young about sex and what sexual responsibility means. Some special dilemmas of adolescents are reviewed in the light of earlier maturing and its consequences. In particular the dangers of sexually transmitted diseases, especially herpes and AIDS, pose some important questions about how we help not only adolescents but younger children to cope with this new disturbing development.

We then face a question which usually goes unexamined, as to what kind of sex education should be available for homosexuals. This is a question normally unasked because sex education is generally perceived as provided by heterosexuals for heterosexuals, with little recognition of the needs of the gay community. Finally we address the need for a new and more satisfactory theory of human sexuality, one which avoids the errors of Freudian theory. We are indebted to Freud and his psychoanalytic successors for many brilliant insights into human nature and its development in the early years. Yet many aspects of his theory of infantile sexuality and the psychosexual development of the young must now be seriously questioned. What is needed is a framework for child-rearing and education which allows us to come to terms with children's sexual growth and help them in it.

14
HELPING ADULTS TO HELP CHILDREN

The two major researches we have reported into children's sexual thinking and children's sexual experiences, together with the survey of expert views, have made clear certain basic facts about sexuality and children. These facts we can summarise as follows.

Children are born sexual and are sexual throughout their development from babyhood through to fully mature adults. They are sexual biologically and physically with all systems ready to go, apart from the reproductive function, which develops gradually until the arrival of adolescence. From a very early age children think about their own and others' sexuality, but soon come up against the stonewalling and evasion of adults. In other words, while biologically sexual children are prevented by our culture (mediated through families, schools and other social institutions) from exploring and finding a meaning through which they can understand and come to terms with their sexuality. We have demonstrated how *à propos* several sexual topics most children are frustrated at not receiving the information which would make sense of their experiences. Their understanding of sex differences is long delayed and confused. They invent garbled and incomplete ideas about babies, how they originate, what happens during pregnancy and how they are born. Sexual intercourse is particularly subject to obscure and evasive explanations, and generally even in these so-called enlightened times modern children are left with some very weird notions which many do not escape from in their adolescent years.

All this implies a long period of deceitfulness with children, often leading to their disillusionment with previously trusted adults. But there are many more fruits of deceit which are detrimental to a child's development.

THE FRUITS OF DECEIT

The first fruit of deceitfulness about sex is the intellectual confusion of children. In most other areas of knowledge we try to enlighten children. In language development, from a child's first weeks of life we talk to them, feeding in words and sentences and by our expressions and actions encouraging babies to begin the first stages of acquiring the meaning of words. We encourage infants to play with blocks and coloured beads so that they develop early concepts of shape, size, colour and number, and so lay the foundations of mathematical meaning. And we support a child's first and successive attempts to master the complex skills needed for them to stand upright, balance and walk. These are but a few examples of how we encourage children to learn and we know that with this encouragement most children become efficient and quick learners.

Not so with sexuality. Far from providing enlightenment we evade, we remain silent, we put children off by saying they are not old enough to understand, we provide partial and misleading information, or we tell downright lies. No wonder children are confused and remain confused about sexuality right into their teenage years. All this results in a retardation in their understanding of sexuality, at a time when they could happily and naturally begin to accept sexuality as part of their nature and everyday life. As in other skills and meanings that children acquire, they need a gradual and encouraging process of explanation and support in their search for sexual meaning.

Another fruit of deceit is a lack of confidence about sexuality which most children betray from an early age. The young are naturally buoyant and resilient beings who thrive when they receive positive support. But when their confidence is undermined they become uncertain and anxious. The evidence we have presented indicates without any doubt how widespread this loss of confidence is. Children are far from confident in talking about sexuality, finding even the basic words for the sex organs 'dirty' and guilt-ridden. In what other area of knowledge are the basic accurate words rejected and substituted for by a childish vocabulary and infantile words which may last a lifetime?

We know from many studies how important it is to build confidence in children so they acquire a positive self-concept, an image of themselves, which serves as a launching pad for activity and exploration. Uncertainty, anxiety, fear, inhibition and guilt are all enemies of a positive self-concept. What kind of image does a young girl build for her feminine future if she thinks at the age of 7 that to have a baby she must be cut open not once but twice? – the first cut to implant the tiny seed or miniature baby in her, and the second to get it out of her body. What happens to the confidence of a boy aged 11 unprepared for his first wet dreams, who is made to feel by cold silence or angry condemnation that he is thoughtless, dirty and immoral?

A third fruit of deceit is the keeping of children at an infantile level not only of thought and emotion but also of status. Much of this is an unconscious process rationalised by the idea that children should retain their childhood innocence as long as possible. This, of course, refers to sexual innocence. From the studies we have presented it can be seen that children are far from 'innocent', since they become increasingly aware of sexuality with increasing age, despite the prevarications of adults. One is reminded of the mythological story of King Canute trying to stem the tide – the action is ineffective and only succeeds in making the King look foolish. This is precisely the reaction of children to adults who deceive them. In their later years they see it as rather stupid of parents and others who have tried to keep them at an infantile level.

Children need increased status as they grow older. We do not talk to infants as we do to babies. Nor do we deal with those in their middle and late childhood as we deal with infants. As children grow in maturity we confer more status, confiding in them more, providing more information, sense and meaning, nourishing their capabilities as they develop. In every other area we try not to keep them immature but we help them forward in their growth. Why should sexuality alone be singled out for arrested development and in some an almost permanent immaturity? These consequences unfortunately continue into adult life, often complicating or destroying adult sexual relationships.

Another fruit of deceit about sexuality is the discouragement of natural curiosity. As we have already noted, this is the most effective spur to children's learning, a feature many schools have not yet harnessed with any success. To blunt the edge of curiosity about sexuality is to render ineffective one of the best tools of learning. And not only does this affect children's search for sexual meaning and its significance, it also undermines their search in other topics. It reduces, as we have seen, the natural self-confidence of children in trying to understand the world around them.

For children to perceive that certain subjects are forbidden or that enquiry is strongly discouraged will impede but not ultimately prevent them from exploring. Far from being totally discouraged they will tend to explore in secret, concealed ways. Children's sexual games probably arise from the less than honest responses and evasions of adults about naming, describing and discussing the sex organs. From being open enquirers in search of truth, children are forced to dissemble and disguise their attempts to know more. Sigmund Freud once wrote that the customary answers given to children about sexual matters damage their 'genuine' instinct for research and as a rule deal the first blow to their confidence in their parents.[1] Deceit by adults breeds distrust and deceit in children.

Finally, one of the most unfortunate fruits of deceit is that children are left unprotected when faced with sexual experiences for which they are unprepared. Ignorance about sexuality leaves children particularly vulnerable in such matters as child sexual abuse. The high percentage we report of children exposed to this danger, especially girls, indicates the gravity of the problem. The evidence is that warnings to children are vague and ineffective unless they have a clear idea of what it is they are being warned about. For example, most of the warnings are based upon the myth of 'stranger danger' when most child sex abusers are known to the children. But vague hints about what may happen will only bewilder children or frighten them about monstrous unnamed harm.

It is a dilemma to know how we can help children view sex in a positive way while warning them that their very sexuality may invite unpleasant attentions from some adults. But in other experiences children learn to differentiate between aspects that are pleasurable, and aspects which may have unpleasant consequences for them. Riding a bicycle gives enormous pleasure and positive confidence for a child, but spills and accidents can be most painful and frightening. To play a game of one's own volition is pleasurable, but to be forced to do so is not. Clearly children can and do make these distinctions and can be taught to do so in sexual matters without destroying their trust in all other human beings.

We have also seen that in preparing girls for the menarche and boys for the first wet dream we cannot delay much beyond the age of 8 or 9 years when for many children pubertal growth will have begun. Perplexing changes are beginning to occur in their bodies, which if unexplained lead to great anxiety and self-consciousness. Much of the embarrassment experienced by young adolescents is because many do not know what is happening, why it is happening and what to do about it. To leave them ignorant and prone to such considerable anxiety is to be thoughtless and negligent. If one duty of adults is to protect children from unfortunate and disturbing experience or prepare them for their future, where sexuality is concerned we stand logic on its head.

ADULTS ARE THE PROBLEM

'It is a problem of our own making; stop hiding sex and there will be no worries about how to reveal it.' So writes Stevi Jackson in her book *Childhood and Sexuality*,[2] putting a view which is supported by the evidence we have presented. Where sex is not hidden, where deceit or silence do not prevail, and where society sets about systematically to communicate information to children through sequential programs, both adults and children have few anxieties. We do not advance Sweden as some kind of social or sexual Utopia but our results reported from Swedish children do indicate positive trends and minimal adult deceit. Swedish children are consistently better informed, less inhibited about discussing sexuality and better prepared for their adolescent and adult lives than their peers in Australia, Britain and North America.

One reason may be that by a long-established tradition of sex education in schools for all children from the age of 7, yesterday's Swedish children have become well equipped parents. It would be inaccurate to say that adult inhibitions about childhood sexuality have disappeared in Sweden, but we can say with some confidence that the situation has improved. Swedish children as they grow into adolescence appear to be more protected from certain sexual dangers, as the figures on teenage pregnancy, teenage venereal diseases and child sexual abuse reveal.[3]

Why do adults in our society have such worries in talking about sexuality with children? Why are adults the problem? We have discussed in the Introduction some reasons why the notion of childhood sexuality is resisted by adults. But human beings do not operate on reason alone. We are all the creatures of our culture and many subscribe to traditional myths about children common in our society. These myths provide perhaps a more profound explanation of why adults have problems about childhood sexuality. They also provide clues about how such problems may be overcome.

'They are only children'

This statement suggests the separateness of children from the adult world and the inference is that we should not treat children as adults. It is true that in modern society we have tended to separate children into a special category. We separate age groups from each other in schools and other institutions so that peer groupings take precedence over family groupings.

But many wrongly interpret the separateness of children as being appropriate because they are immature, because of their absorption in play, and their lack of seriousness about matters concerning the adult world, as though they are creatures of another world. What this myth fails to recognise is that children of any age are part of a gradual process of development and that they have similar if not identical human qualities to grown-ups. By emphasising that they are diminutive, we ensure that their status, rights, curiosity, needs and potential are diminished. To assert 'They are only children' is to relegate them to a lesser world where important matters, such as sexuality, are too great a burden for children to bear.

Another facet of this view is that childhood is a carefree period of life which children should be left to enjoy as long as possible. Serious matters, such as sex, should not intervene, and their innocence should be left uncontaminated until enlightenment is absolutely necessary.

What we have argued is precisely the opposite. Children are not innocent of sexuality or sexual knowledge and a true under-standing of sexuality is a long and complex process too serious to be left until adolescence. Childhood is not the carefree period of life sentimentalists suggest it to be; it has its anxieties and problems about which we must help children. And they are not lesser beings, but individuals of worth, at whatever stage of development they may be, individuals whose needs are to be met and who have distinctive rights.

'Sexuality is for adults only'

This is an extension of the first myth but it is based primarily on a narrow and incorrect definition of sexuality (sexuality for adults as bedroom sexuality, which is fundamentally based upon sexual reproduction). The argument then is that children cannot be reproductive until their adolescence (a fact not entirely true) and therefore education in sexuality can be delayed until such time as they have to face bedroom or reproductive activities.

This argument is circular and self-defeating. How can the young learn to be responsible or experienced without being given responsibility and encountering experience as they grow? And it founders on the obvious fact that sex and sexuality are far more than reproduction, consisting of a vast number of experiences, as we have already illustrated, encountered throughout childhood. This adult myth is based upon the fallacy that sexuality suddenly begins in adolescence and no semblance of it appears before that time.

Our society tries to assert a monopoly of sexuality for adults in many ways. We grade certain kinds of films as suitable for adults only. Books for children tend to be sexless apart from the distinction among its characters of boys and girls, and men and women. Children's dolls are usually without genitals or nipples. And almost the entire adult world, until recently, has entered into a conspiracy of silence. The fact that we have delayed sex education programs, when we allow them at all, until the secondary school stage is also an assertion that preparation for sex should not begin until adolescence. Getting sex education in primary schools is still a major battle to be fought in many areas, despite the obvious developmental facts of early maturing now becoming known.

Sexuality is a feature of all human life from the cradle to the grave. Children need to be inducted and educated into their own sexuality from their early years. It is entirely unrealistic to expect children to inhibit interests and conceal experiences of their own sex organs, the growth of their own bodies and their curiosity about the adult world of sexuality around them. Marriage, babies, abortions, divorces are some of the topics which the media, especially television, thrust into their consciousness, as well as the subjects of love-making and reproduction.

'They are too young to understand'

This is an extension of the second myth, for it is argued that children have no capacity to understand its complexity, with which even adults may have difficulty. Adults frequently defer their answers to children's sexual questions with the remark 'Wait until you're old enough to understand, dear.' Our own researches reported in this book and the research of others expose this as a falsehood. Yet it is so often used as an excuse to delay that we shall deal with this myth in some detail.

We have demonstrated that children from an early age are quite capable of understanding most sexual matters which affect them. This depends, of course, upon simple explanations and reasonably clear information being given. We found a number of children between 5 and 7 years of quite average ability able to tell us about sex differences, using the right names of sex organs, how babies originate through some kind of sexual joining, how babies are born and many other details. While these were the exceptions, it demonstrates that for children who are given sensible explanations in the early years there is no conceptual difficulty in grasping basic sexual facts. We did find two areas which appear to have intrinsic difficulties for the very young. One of these was how the sex of a baby is determined at birth, since grasping the details of genes and chromosomes is a fairly complex matter. The other is how the embryo, fetus and baby evolve as living beings, a process which is unseen and difficult for children to comprehend. Sex determination seems best left to secondary schooling, but the development of a baby during pregnancy can be dealt with earlier using pictures and diagrams.

The responses of the Swedish children interviewed in our research, compared with their English-speaking peers, provide strong evidence that children have the intellectual capacity to deal with most sexual information. The problem is not intellectual limitation, but being kept uninformed, or worse, misinformed by partial explanations complicated by the embarrassments and inhibitions of adults.

It is true that children can be confused by too much information. As in any other subject they need simple ideas to begin with, gradually increasing in detail and complexity. This is what sound school syllabuses try to do, by providing a sequence of topics, graded by age, so that children become familiar with the language and concepts needed to build up a comprehensive picture and what it all means. This is the way children are introduced to mathematics, geography, reading, history and nature study.

Because many adults are worried about sexuality, they often try to deal with 'the facts of life' in one session. More than one parent has then heaved a sigh of relief and been heard to say 'Thank goodness that's over'. It is self-evident that to do this with any other topic would result in mental indigestion. We accept the gradual graded approach in most matters, returning to basic details which children do not fully grasp at first, then providing more advanced ideas. Sexuality is like any other topic, requiring the same educational process, and no one-off treatment can deal with it satisfactorily.

Many children we interviewed at the age of 7 had an intelligent grasp of what sexuality is and how it affects themselves. By 9 years many knew what would happen to their bodies during puberty and understood the basic facts about reproduction. All these children appeared to share several experiences in common:

- parents who explained matters simply to them when the children asked questions;
- parents who used family experiences such as bathtime or the expectation of a new baby to talk about what was happening and what it all meant;
- adults, including teachers, who systematically explained to growing children sexual matters they were curious about, repeating information several times.

'If you tell them about sex they will go out and do it'

Parents in particular are scared by this kind of assertion. It evokes worries, often unconsciously felt, that sex is some kind of pollutant from which they must protect their children. They would rather their children were kept in ignorance than exposed to sexual temptation. It is a myth used to delay or prevent sex education in schools, based upon the fear of stimulating precocious sexual relations among the young.

Evidence about increased sexual activities of the young came to public notice long before sex education was ever introduced into schools, starting with World War I and accelerating after World War II. As Schofield points out, it is adults not children who created the permissive society over several generations.[4] Figures for sexual 'delinquency' such as teenage pregnancy are far greater in countries which restrict or delay sex education such as the USA, Italy, Thailand and New Zealand. Conversely those countries which once had high rates of teenage sexual problems but which introduced earlier and comprehensive sex education in schools witnessed after ten years a dramatic decrease in these figures. Examples of this are Sweden and Denmark.

Cause and effect are difficult to determine but systematic introduction to 'the facts of life' would appear to protect children from so-called temptation rather than encourage greater sexual activity. There is further American evidence to show that where parents play a part in the sex education of their own children, such children are less likely to engage in early sexual intercourse.[5]

Studies carried out with teenage girls who become pregnant also show them to be ignorant not only about contraception but about conception. In other words it is the ignorant who are at greater risk, not the informed.

Overall it appears that it is not sex information whether given in the home or in school which stimulates full sexual activity among the young. It is other factors such as external influences of a sexy, sex-obsessed and sexually stimulating society which arouse the young, together with internal factors such as hormonal growth and an earlier adolescence. Knowledge tends to protect.

'You cannot teach children about responsible sex until they are much older'

This myth is an extension of the view that children are not old enough to understand sexuality. Since their grasp of moral values in general is limited it is therefore argued that children cannot be morally responsible where sex is concerned. Since they cannot handle it, it is dangerous to teach them about it.

Mythologies do contain some elements of truth and it must be recognised that moral development is a slow and gradual process. What we refer to as moral values, that is, the standards of right and wrong we try to live by, are not fully formulated or acted upon until mid-adolescence or even later. Even some adults do not appear to possess moral values, other than by accepting the conventions of their society.

Children nevertheless do develop a morality from an early age and begin to judge what is right and wrong. This may start with a primitive morality of fear, simply the avoidance of actions which incur painful consequences such as punishment. They may then progress to a morality based upon external authority, whereby something is right or wrong because powerful adults say it is so. A move forward is towards the morality of convention created by public opinion, an influence older children and adolescents feel particularly through peer pressures. The evidence is that few move to the highest level of individually held moral values which guide their behaviour, in sexual and in other matters.[6] Fully grown adults, who are usually judged to be responsible for their actions, may behave at any one of these moral levels, acting from fear, authoritarian influence, peer pressure or personally held moral values. Very few behave at a consistently high level of morality.

So it is with children. They respond to suggestions that it is wrong to indulge in masturbatory activities in public. They easily recognise that some sexual matters will offend or distress other people. They soon learn that other children have rights as well as themselves, and that it is wrong to hurt or damage them. Naturally they make mistakes, but moral learning depends upon learning from one's mistakes and understanding the moral implications and consequences involved in one's actions.

The fear behind this myth is again the fear of premature copulation, that the young may get involved in reproductive activities before they can handle such an experience. The evidence is that earlier experience and understanding of sexuality is well within the moral competence of children. Yet not all sexual matters need to be dealt with in a moral context. What is there moral about recognising realistically one's sexual identity as a girl or boy? What ethical considerations enter into knowing about how a baby is born? What is appropriate behaviour when a girl copes with her first menstruation is more physical necessity than a moral matter.

We have already noted the need for the modesty training of children where nakedness is concerned, for some guidance, not necessarily moral, regarding masturbation and hints on how sexual behaviour with other children can be handled. Children may also have to face sexual interference by adults. In all these sexual experiences, children will usually behave as responsibly as they have been taught. To delay helping children in these matters until they are morally mature is totally unrealistic, just as it is absurd to make a similar demand of all adults.

In reviewing the five major myths that adults apply to children, it must be recognised that myths, however untrue they may be, have a powerful hold on the human mind. It has been said that myths may be more powerful than reality in determining attitudes and decisions. At best a myth contains a half-truth and at its worst a total falsehood. It is a necessary first step to see the adult myths we have received for what they are, as we have done in this chapter. But because they demonstrate that we in the adult world are the problem, more positive approaches are required. What are these positive approaches and how can adults help children to deal with sexuality?

WHAT CHILDREN NEED FROM ADULTS

Sex education begins at an early age. Even if parents say little or nothing, whether they recognise it or not, whether they like it or not, they are their children's first sex educators. The evidence is clear that by the age of 5, children have learned sexual language or how to avoid it as involving shameful dirty words. They have begun to explore sexuality naturally and unself-consciously, or have learned to inhibit their curiosity in this area. Their first sexual experiences of touching their own sexual organs have either been accepted and dealt with in a positive way, or they have learned in no uncertain manner the undesirability of such behaviour. Children may have had to deal with adults who have a wholesome healthy view of sex, or with those who subscribe to misleading myths about childhood sexuality.

We shall examine what young children in particular need if they are to enjoy a healthy sexual development. What goes for the very young may also serve as guidelines suitable for older children, and they also apply to the period of pubertal growth and ensuing adolescence.

The acceptance of sexuality in infancy and childhood

Children need adults around them, parents in particular, who have come to terms with the fact that they are sexual throughout babyhood, infancy and later childhood. Such adults do not deceive themselves that sexuality is something that begins to emerge during adolescence or is mysteriously reserved for adults only. It is part of a continuous process from birth, indeed from the moment of conception. Not to recognise it is akin to a refusal to accept a child's basic appetite for food, or the natural activities of crawling and walking.

Accepting a child's developing sexuality is more than mere toleration of it. Many of us as adults have not learned to accept the naturalness of sex, and still have difficulties being open about it as a topic. We are the products of our own childhood, the inhibitions and repressions of our own upbringing and the shortcomings of our parents' inhibitions and hangups. Yet such a repetitive and negative cycle can be broken, as the experiences of several Scandinavian countries show. Within a generation or two of sex education programs being introduced, future parents began to be more understanding and accepting of sexuality in general, and their own sexuality in particular. This in turn was conveyed to their own children so that over a period a more positive attitude to sexuality began to prevail. Despite attacks from the bigoted and the fearful, a de-mythologising process occurred and in those countries a more accepting climate has been established.

Why should these countries be more progressive than other countries in these matters? The major reasons appear to be a national commitment to a sound socially directed education system and also the belief that what experts say should be translated into policy. So, for example, the Swedish National Board of Education took seriously what their commission on sex education, made up of experts as well as community representatives, reported on childhood and adolescent trends. Consequently a new syllabus appeared in the mid-1970s based upon research, specifically to face such facts as earlier sexual maturing and earlier sexual activity.

Denigraters of Scandinavian societies have been vocal in Australia, Britain and America, describing them as cesspools of iniquity, encouragers of pedophilia and childhood pornography. Such attacks are ill informed and simply peddle new misleading mythologies by quoting or misusing distorted statistics. Overall the picture is one of more accepting, open and honest societies where the sexual problems of the young have decreased. Teenage pregnancies, venereal infections and other difficulties still exist, but they are measurably less than elsewhere.

What then does an acceptance of childhood sexuality mean? One thing it does not mean is to encourage the young to 'have sex'. On the contrary it distinguishes between developing sexuality and reproductive sexuality. Preparing for reproductive sexuality eventually is not to condone or encourage it before the young can exercise sound judgment and responsible behaviour, as we have previously noted.

Acceptance of sexuality in childhood by adults means a recognition of its inevitability, namely that the curiosity of children about their own bodies and the bodies of others is natural. It means acknowledging that children have a right to know and to explore without condemnation, and indeed require the support of adults in their search for meaning.

Many of us may be intellectually accepting of these facts but still feel emotionally uncomfortable with them. This difficulty is shared possibly by the majority of adults in our society. For the good of our children we have to live with such discomfort. Indeed, we may live the rest of our lives with such inhibitions. We can only hope that by our own courage our children will feel more comfortable with sex and more accepting of their children in turn.

Sensitive handling of sexual limits

Children need adults who recognise that a child's sexuality does not occur within a single family but takes place in a wider social context. We may be accepting of our own children's sexuality and develop family traditions of openness. Yet there may well be disapproving neighbours, whose children are our children's playmates, who may react adversely to our ideas. Visitors, especially elderly relatives, may be embarrassed by the comments and activities of our children, who do not initially distinguish between what is acceptable within the confines of the close-knit family and what is unacceptable outside it.

While neighbours, relatives and others should not be allowed to dictate what we should do in rearing our children, we must help the young to make some social distinctions. This is what we call the sensitive handling of sexual limits, helping children understand what the limits are and when they should be applied. We cannot avoid all embarrassments in advance but we can ensure that a child is aware of possible difficulties. For example, a little girl who announces to a visiting elderly aunt 'My brother's got a penis and I haven't' may be unaware of the shocked atmosphere such a statement produces. Maybe in the circumstances it will be best to leave it undiscussed but it can provide later an opportunity for helping this child be more sensitive in the future.

For those who want to be more open and accepting this poses a dilemma. But children have to live in a real world and have to adjust to the need for sexual limits. Many modern families resolve the dilemma, being open and accepting of sexuality within the family but educating their children realistically about the pressures and difficulties of other people. When neighbours complain about your child using dirty language in playing with their children, when in fact they used the correct names for the sex organs, that is a matter between adults which may be handled without rebuke or reprimand of the child concerned. But in the shocked elderly relative incident it would be wise to say 'Remember Aunt Edna is much older and isn't used to such talk. It's all right in the family but not with visitors, unless they talk about it.' Such advice to children is a necessary part of their social education.

It is not only with adults that restraints are needed. Some limitations can be discussed about what children do in their play with one another. The root cause of sexual curiosity about the sex organs can be removed or minimised if children know from an early age what they look like, what they are for and what they are called. But sensitive advice is needed about not hurting another child, or not allowing another child to hurt a playmate. Because children may feel threatened, hurt or frightened they should be taught how to deal with such situations. Again there is a dilemma in anticipating these experiences and at the same time not introducing unnecessary fears or imagined horrors. The sensitive parent or teacher learns to handle this according to the needs and development of individual children.

Honesty the best policy

Children need adults around them who are honest about sexuality. We have noted what the fruits of sexual deceit with children are: confusion, lack of confidence, infantile responses, and the discouragement of natural curiosity. More importantly, dishonesty leaves children unprepared for and unprotected from the sexual predators and other dangers to which they are exposed.

Honest adults answer children's questions and build up a relationship of trust which avoidance, prevarication, half-truths or silence can destroy. The process of answering children's questions is not always easy. Initially it means overcoming our own embarrassments and discomforts on the subject, not an easy task for many of us. If we are uncertain what kind of questions will be thrown at us, often at the most unlikely moments, or how to answer them, there are many books which can provide help.[7]

One aspect of being honest about sexuality is admitting with some questions that we don't know. Some questions, particularly from older children, may not be readily answered and no one expects you to be a walking sexual encyclopedia. It is useful to have a few books which can provide answers, both at home and at school, so that one can say 'I don't know the answer to that one, but let's look it up.' Such an open approach is entirely honest and also encourages a child to use books to get information, especially if such books are on the open shelves, readily accessible.

But many parents have reported to us that they have prepared themselves to answer questions and then been dismayed that the questions do not come. It may be, of course, that children have received messages by body language and other communications that the topic of sexuality is an embarrassing one. It may not have been parents who have communicated this, but peers and other adults who have signalled taboos, disapproval and negativisms, which have then inhibited the questions which would naturally arise.

If such is the case, it is vital to raise certain sexual topics with children to indicate to them that you do not share the negative views which they may have encountered. Such topics as the sex organs can be casually discussed during bathtimes, the origins of babies when a pregnancy occurs, the physical changes in boys and girls, and men and women, as children begin to enter the first stages of puberty. Both casually and systematically, adults can indicate by this introduction of sexual matters that they are askable adults.

Another aspect of honesty is the readiness to use correct names, and the avoidance of coy or misleading explanations or of words such as 'seed' and 'egg', when 'sperm' and 'ovum' are far better. These may require some initial explanation but in the long run are clearer terms to use and they tend to avoid mythological confusions. Many adults, especially with younger children, may limit their answers to partial explanations according to the myth that the children are too young to understand. While long, technical and complex answers are to be avoided, it appears to be better to tell more rather than less. Children will take what they can from an answer and ignore what they cannot understand. Our research has indicated that adults tend to seriously underestimate the capacity of children to understand in the area of sexuality. On the other hand, there is clear evidence that explanations need repeating and elaborating as children grow older, so that they become familiar with the language and concepts of sexuality. Sexuality is a complex topic and as we have already noted cannot be dismissed in a single talk or lecture on 'the facts of life'. Systematised and gradually acquired knowledge is required, as in all other subjects.

Home-based sex education is not enough

While parents are the first and probably in some cases the child's best sex educators, the evidence is overwhelming that most parents sidestep their responsibilities in this regard. It will be many decades before it can be claimed with any confidence that home-based sex education exists at a suitable level for most children.

In Australia a 1982 study revealed that 80% of teenagers claimed no significant sex information was communicated by parents. In America a well-based report revealed that many parents wish to teach their children about sex but feel incapable of it. Schofield's report on the English scene showed that 66% of boys and 25% of girls received no sex information from parents. But even those who did receive help from their parents stated that it was only partial and provided only haphazard and intermittent support.

Plainly children, and their parents as well, need more than the home can provide. While clubs, churches and other organisations might provide some further support, there appears to be no substitute for systematic teaching about sex and human relations in our schools. Since children seem to have no say in what they are to be taught, they need adults to speak for them and request from schools a suitable curriculum in this topic.

We make no apologies for repeating this need, since the evidence is overwhelming and the problem is a most urgent one. And there have to be enough educators and politicians of courage to press for more provision and at the appropriate levels beginning in the primary (elementary) school. Parents too can apply continuous pressure on local schools and through the press to see that sex education is provided. Otherwise we shall go from one generation to the next, denying children the training they should receive as future parents so that they can become better parents than the previous generations.

Sexuality is the concern of the whole of society, and it is through its social agencies, particularly the schools, that sure but gradual changes can be accomplished. If sexuality as currently handled produces grave social problems and renders large sections of the population unhappy, frustrated and unfulfilled, the remedies lie in our hands. We must start at the beginning, with our children, the future generation of parents.

15
SOME DIFFICULT AND UNRESOLVED ISSUES

We have tried to provide some clear guidelines for parents, teachers and other care-givers and educators, so they can understand and handle child sexuality. We believe the findings of research are a surer foundation than folklore and myths about children. Yet some issues are not so simply resolved since many of them involve personal and social matters of a complex kind. Rather than confuse by introducing these complexities earlier we have left them to this final chapter so they can be seen against the overall picture we have presented.

No child is exactly the same as another, not even identical twins who share exactly the same genetic inheritance, for even identical twins have different experiences as they grow up and develop different personalities. Each child is a unique combination of physical inheritance and interactions with the environment which between them stimulate an individual's intellectual, social and behavioural development. Sexuality is no exception to this. We have pointed out the wide varieties in sexual development during infancy and childhood, the speed of growth and the fact that some children are early and others are late maturers. While most children display an early interest in sexual matters, there are some for whom such interest is only peripheral and of little consequence. Most children explore sexuality through games with friends, but there are others who seem to exhibit no such curiosity. Certainly some children, as do some adults, possess a stronger sexual drive than others.

Despite this wide range of differences, all fall within what we describe as normal, and do not invalidate the generalisations we have made so far. However, parents and teachers who have

235

to deal with the young daily need to translate these generalisations into what is suitable for individual children.

One dilemma often expressed is that of dealing with children of disparate ages in a family, or a mixture of children in a school class. We can be paralysed by uncertainty, wondering whether what we present to help early developers may in some way be premature for those slow in their pubertal development. This dilemma is more imagined than real. Children who are younger, less able intellectually or slow physical developers will gain a great deal from early discussions and explanations about sexuality, even if they do not comprehend all that is said. And even if much seems to go over their heads, they experience a much-needed assurance that sex is not a taboo subject and that it can be looked at calmly in the normal course of discussion and conversation. They cannot be harmed if they hear the basic biological facts of sexuality and their meaning discussed many times during their childhood. Indeed, they stand to benefit by a deeper understanding and by acquiring more positive attitudes.

Another dilemma is often posed by differences between families, where family traditions, expectations and behaviours will certainly not be identical with those of neighbours or parents of children attending the same school. In most countries, Australia in particlar, the multiplicity of cultures, ethnic origins and religions is very evident. We then face a diversity of values, moral judgments and sexual attitudes, not all of which are compatible with each other. We shall begin with this problem, since it affects individual families and especially school-based sex education programs.

VALUES AND MORALS IN SEXUAL TEACHING

There are two aspects to this problem of what to teach in terms of sexual values to the young. The first is the dilemma of individual families whose values, determined by their ethnic, religious and cultural backgrounds, may appear to be opposed to a greater openness, greater honesty and even acceptance of some sexual characteristics we have described as normal. The second is the dilemma faced by teachers and schools who are well aware of the differing and apparently incompatible values held by the many families who form their clientele. If a state school sex education program is to be provided, how can the views of born-again Christian, Humanist, Roman Catholic, Jewish Orthodox and Muslim parents be catered for? Many of these groups have quite specific views on such matters as masturbation, sex before marriage, divorce, contraception, abortion and the status of girls.

At the outset, whether looked at from a parent's viewpoint or from the question of school provision, it must be said that no sexual teaching can be separated from values and morality. Some sexual matters such as sex differences, the facts of human growth, how to educate a girl for her first menstruation may all appear to be objectively based on fact. But what one teaches about sex and how it is taught is invariably within some kind of moral framework, whether consciously formulated or not. In asserting that sex is a normal and healthy human activity, a viewpoint shared by many, we may run contrary to certain theological views of original sin and the demonic nature of children, or the Freudian view of the destructive nature of the Id.

In the public mind also, morality and sexual restraint are often seen as identical. Sex is viewed as a basic animal drive to be controlled, and the inculcation of moral values, teaching what is right and wrong, is seen as an essential task of sex education. This is the view of many who demand that sex education should emphasise traditional moral values.

The situation we have outlined poses a dilemma for parents and schools alike. If morality and sex are inseparable, if values make up an important part of teaching about sex, what kind of morality and values should we be teaching? What is meant by traditional moral values and what should be done if we cannot share them as individuals, families, schools or communities? Should we distinguish between education for moral choice and moral indoctrination?

In its latest syllabus the Swedish Ministry of Education addresses these questions.[1] The latest manual provides some clear and refreshing guidelines which endorse the view that in sex education moral values should be taught, particularly with adolescents. The objective is not moral indoctrination but helping the young make informed moral choices. Despite the fact that 94% of the Swedish population is Lutheran, there are considerable numbers from Turkey, Cyprus and North Africa who come to Sweden as guest-workers. Many of these are not only non-Christian but are followers of the religion of Islam.

Since all children must receive sex education in Swedish schools, they are taught on the following moral basis. First, the program is based upon widely accepted community values relating to sexuality. Second, where there are conflicting values, all conflicting views are to be taught as objectively and impartially as possible. The Swedes take the view that since no democratic educational system can justify teaching one exclusive set of moral values, then there is no alternative to presenting them all. What specifically the Swedes recommend is worth examining in some detail, for it provides answers to the various moral questions we have raised.

The Swedish manual states that there are basic common values held by practically all in Swedish communities. In sexual matters these include the centrality of love, caring, respect, responsibility and fidelity. These common values are elaborated in terms of consequences which older students especially can understand. For example it is asserted that

- sexual responsibility is incompatible with unwanted pregnancies, the need for abortion or adoption, and transmission of disease;
- the right to sexual privacy implies that sexual experience by force is a violation;
- sexuality as an expression of a personal relationship is preferable to impersonal casual experiences for the purpose of sexual gratification;
- faithfulness between couples is more than refraining from sexual intercourse with a third person, but is an expression of commitment to a broader relationship;
- both sexes have equal rights which involve the rejection of double standards for males and traditional sex roles and sex stereotypes;
- rights imply the rejection of racial or ethnic discrimination, the acceptance of homosexuality, restoring the sexual

rights of the physically and mentally handicapped, inmates of prisons, the elderly and others.

An interesting rider is clearly stated, that where individuals or minorities wish to violate community values (as when many Muslims resist sexual equality and object to girls being taught such values) the majority view must prevail, the Swedes asserting that the rights of children are paramount.

As well as basic community values which have majority public support and approval, values held by different groups, religious bodies or ethnic minorities are to be taught, 'objectively and impartially'. Teachers are enjoined to be truthful and sensitive in such matters, so that children can understand the various moral viewpoints expressed in Swedish society. Most countries would identify with the topics the Swedes list as 'controversial'. These are

- Abortion: here two conflicting values need to be clarified – one, that from conception each child is a human being, and the other that every pregnant woman is entitled to bear her child or not.
- Contraception: this is viewed by some as a responsible precaution to conceive only wanted children in contrast to the opposing religious views about the primary purpose of sexual intercourse. 'Natural' as well as artificial methods of birth control are to be taught.
- Premarital relations: these are not accepted by some but for others are acceptable.
- Ex-nuptial children: in Sweden these are accepted by the government as 'legitimate' but are disapproved of by some religious groups.
- Chastity: the official view is that, especially because of earlier maturing, chastity should be recommended, but where not accepted the young should be prepared with contraceptive advice.

Divorce, masturbation and homosexuality, about which certain religious bodies have specific views, are also controversial.

The Swedes appear to have adopted a sensible solution to a problem which threatens in many countries to prevent or disrupt school-based sex education. Charges of immoral or 'liberal' teaching are used by militant minorities who wish to indoctrinate the young with their particular moral code. If all moral views are presented, these objections are seen to have no substance.

For parents the problem is more personal than for school authorities devising syllabuses. But the situation for parents has some similarities with that of the school. While by teaching and example we teach children our own values about sex, we cannot shield them from contradictory values. It is wise for parents to recognise that their children will hear these contrary views and to openly discuss them in the course of normal family life. Ultimately children, during their adolescent years especially, will make up their own minds. Better to prepare them for the choices they will have to make by providing them with informed and wise guidance than to leave them informed of only one viewpoint, however passionately we may hold that viewpoint ourselves.

SOME SPECIAL DILEMMAS OF ADOLESCENTS

We have highlighted certain trends which intensify the problems of those who are concerned with adolescents. As revealed by research these trends are
- earlier physical and sexual maturing;
- earlier sexual activity, including earlier first intercourse;
- earlier vulnerability to sexually transmitted diseases;
- earlier proneness to teenage pregnancy;
- comparative ignorance of teenagers about contraception and sexually transmitted diseases;
- the probability of not using contraceptives in first sexual experiences.

However shocked we may be about these trends they do intensify the problems involved in deciding what we shall advise children and adolescents about such matters and when we should begin to give the advice.

While these trends have been evident for a long time, there are new features which seem to demand a reappraisal of what and when we should teach the young about sexuality. The most recent and urgent development is the growing awareness of incurable sexual diseases, and particularly the spread of AIDS (Acquired Immune Deficiency Syndrome) which can kill. It has been known for some time, although the general public has not been particularly well informed, that some other sexually transmitted diseases are incurable. These include certain types of hepatitis and herpes, but this list now includes AIDS with the additional threat of a possible early death.

Deaths from AIDS have resulted from addicts sharing needles, anal intercourse by both heterosexuals and homosexuals, vaginal intercourse with an infected partner and in some cases blood transfusions from infected donors. As recent information on the media has indicated, heterosexuals as well as homosexuals are at risk, particularly if they have sex with numerous partners. Advertisements by health authorities have stressed two matters, the need to confine sex to one partner, and the need to use condoms as the most reliable means of avoiding infection. These advertisements, similar in many English-speaking countries, may well frighten large numbers of people into celibacy or into an exclusive sexual relationship or the use of condoms as a precaution. For adults dealing with adolescents, however, this poses two dilemmas. First, when shall we tell the young about these dangers, and second, what precise information is appropriate?

Before we address these questions, it will be useful to rehearse the basic facts of the sexual trends we have summarised.

The average age of girls' first menstruation in Australia is between 12 and 12½ years of age, and for boys' first wet dreams about 12 to 13 years. If this is the average then a considerable number mature between 10 and 12 years, a few earlier than that. Interest in sexual activity therefore comes earlier and our figures of first intercourse (as reported in Chapter 13) show that 8% occurs at 13 years or below and 39% between 14 and 16 years. These figures include the small but still disconcerting numbers of those who are the victims of certain kinds of child sexual abuse, the peak years for which are between 8 and 11. All this indicates the vulnerability of the young to possible sexual infection at a much younger age than the general public wishes to believe.

Add to these facts, the demonstrable ignorance of teenagers

about contraception, and their lack of interest in and knowledge about sexually transmitted diseases, and we can see how vulnerable are the young. The most widely understood contraceptive is the pill, but while this offers protection from pregnancy it is not so widely known that it does not protect from disease. All the evidence is that boys, if sexually active, are reluctant to use a condom and assume birth control should be left to the girls. Here we have a recipe for sexual disaster among the young of possibly increasing dimensions.

These facts lead us to the inescapable conclusion that information about these dangers and how to avoid them cannot be left later than 9 or 10 years of age, that is towards the top age groups in primary schools. But another feature becomes increasingly clear, that nothing can be understood about sexually transmitted disease without a grasp of the basic biology of sex, of sexual joining, of the nature of sperm and how it is transmitted from male to female. As in dealing with child sexual abuse, a special AIDS program for 9-year-olds will be ineffective unless seen within a broader understanding of sexuality. In other words, general sex education must lay the foundations for understanding the words and concepts involved in specific programs. This incidentally involves parents, especially where primary schools are slow to provide sex education.

If then we begin this general program with children no older than say 9, what shall we teach? This creates a dilemma for those who argue for retaining the sexual innocence of children. It also poses a dilemma for those who want to rear their children into a happy, positive view of sex. If horror responses to AIDS advertisements screened on Australian television are the major impact, as some of the public have criticised, does not this destroy positive attitudes to sexuality and substitute fear and distrust? The proponents of such advertisements say that the public needs to be startled out of its complacency about AIDS by shock tactics emphasising that the consequences are death as well as disease.

What then shall we begin to teach 9-year-olds to help them face their present situation and their pubertal development into adolescence, with its attendant dangers? Here is what the evidence indicates are the major facts they need to know:

242

- the nature of sexuality as seen in boys and girls and men and women;
- the correct names of both the male and female sex organs;
- the various uses of the sex organs, the primary ones being sexual intercourse both for pleasure and the begetting of children;
- an emphasis upon sexual activity based upon love, respect, caring and trust, and the delaying of such experience until such a relationship develops;
- the dangers of casual sexual intercourse in terms of teenage pregnancy and sexually transmitted diseases;
- how to avoid teenage pregnancy by (1) abstaining from sex (2) using contraceptives, to be specified in detail with some explanations about how they work;
- how to avoid sexually transmitted diseases by (1) abstaining from sex (2) using one particular kind of contraceptive, namely a condom.

All these facts and associated ideas are well within the conceptual grasp of average 9-year-olds, if put simply. For 10- and 11-year-olds the facts should be given again, with more detailed information. For 12- and 13-year-olds, repetition is still needed, with greater emphasis upon responsible sex, the need for a satisfying relationship and the importance of fidelity.

There is, however, a major social choice which society must make if the sexual drives of some lead to full sexual intercourse. This is whether to make contraceptives available to the young not only in pharmacies but in slot machines in public places. It is a contradiction if advice is given on how to avoid pregnancy and disease and the means of such avoidance are denied.

These basic recommendations will be accepted by most people as sensible. Some, however, will find parts of them controversial, as might committed Roman Catholics to information about artificial means of birth control. Catholic and other religious schools, as well as individual religious parents, still have to work out what is consistent with their faith and with the protection of their children. Religious belief alone is not a sufficient safeguard from the sexual dangers which threaten the young today.

One thing is clear. If we are to prepare adolescents for the sexual choices they have to make, we cannot leave it to the time of adolescence itself to begin. We have to start during childhood to prepare them intellectually, emotionally and morally to cope with their own sexuality and the temptations they will soon face.

THE SEX EDUCATION OF HOMOSEXUALS

In reviewing the facts about homosexual experiences in the teenage years (in Chapter 13) we reported that some 10% of the population is homosexual. In our view this is a conservative estimate, depending on whether the definition includes those who are bisexual, those who are in a practising homosexual relationship and proclaim themselves gay, and those who are only occasionally so. A broader definition would lead to estimates of one in five of the population. In any school class of thirty, this would mean between three and six students who will at some time be involved in homosexual experiences.

This is a considerable proportion of any human group and the heterosexual majority of the population, especially parents and teachers, have to come to terms with this. Sex education (where provided in schools) tends to be planned for hetero-sexuals, to be taught by heterosexuals to groups assumed to be heterosexuals. Given the fact that, as Michael Carrera has said, 'Homosexuality is not a choice people make', this places some people in an educational dilemma. How should the topic of homosexuality be dealt with in schools? Will it be seen as the promotion of homosexuality? Is society ready for such a step and if it is, are there special needs of those children who will prefer their own sex during their adolescent and adult years?

These questions may well disturb those in the present climate who accuse homosexuals of being primarily responsible for the spread of AIDS, using this as a justification for labelling homosexuality as a perversion. We subscribe to neither of these opinions, since the facts appear not to support them. Thinking and sensitive citizens need to address those questions. We our-selves raise them simply because we have met many troubled parents, after we have talked about sex education at parent–teacher gatherings, who have raised similar queries. These are parents who have discovered that a child of theirs is gay. Their attitudes vary from 'What did I do wrong?' to 'What can I do to help my child?'

The facts of the matter are that being gay is not usually a person's choice, that parents should not blame themselves and it is more constructive to ask the more positive question, how can we help such children?

In the past parents and teachers have tried various strategies which have proved unsuccessful and usually resulted in unhappiness for all parties concerned. To condemn a person for same-sex preferences is purely destructive. To try to dissuade gays from being gay and encourage a pretence of being 'normal', that is heterosexual, may be similarly destructive. Worst of all is to refer a child for psychiatric treatment, as some parents do, as though being gay were some kind of sickness or gross perversion. What is required is a more positive approach based upon what the needs are of that proportion of the young who will develop same-sex preferences.

We do not advocate a separate form of sex education, since it will not be evident until the ages of thirteen or fourteen at the earliest who are the future gays. What we do recommend is that homosexuality as a topic be included in all sex education programs in such a way that all children, future heterosexuals as well as homosexuals, gain a clear picture of what being gay involves, its normality for a certain proportion of the population, and the difficulties and dangers which gays have to face. We cover these characteristics when dealing with heterosexuality, so why not for homosexuals? Many societies have rescinded laws which make homosexual activity a criminal offence, although anomalies and prejudices still remain. Educational authorities responsible for curriculum guidelines have shown themselves to be nervous about including this topic in syllabuses. But natural justice and the needs of future gays require us to be more courageous and constructive about such matters.

If we were to include positive approaches in our sex education courses, within a generation or two we would largely diminish if not eradicate the hostilities and prejudices which most homosexuals encounter. There will probably always be small groups of ill-informed bigots who continue to be loud in their condemnation, but their influence should not determine what is best for our children.

Even where the topic of homosexuality is included in sex education provision, it is often dealt with as the acceptance of an aberration, gays still being seen as abnormal or queers. What this does is maybe to educate heterosexuals into less condemnatory attitudes, but it does not help the self-image and self-respect of a gay boy or lesbian girl of the future. Just as the information about masturbation that 'you are not the only one' brings immense relief for adolescents, so the knowledge that many have same-sex preferences will relieve future gays of unnecessary anxieties. They will have difficulties enough without adding to their problems.

It will help also if they know how to contact those who are more supportive, where they can receive information and advice. All sex books designed for adolescents should contain telephone numbers and addresses where gay groups can be reached.[2] In most large cities these are listed in the telephone book under 'Gay' or 'Gayline'. It is also important for young gays, especially in the present climate of crisis, to be able to get such publications as *Safe Sex*, published by gay groups on the topic of AIDS.

Parents, teachers and those who may be involved in giving advice to the young on these matters should seek out information for themselves so they can be fully informed about homosexuality.[3]

The hysteria about gays in the late 1980s generated by the spread of AIDS has resurrected many of the prejudices and myths which were beginning to recede. We predict that this hysteria will die away as facts take the place of mythologies and that we will continue to move slowly to a greater acceptance of same-sex preferences as a valid lifestyle. It is significant that lesbian choices have already received wider acceptance in the community. What is needed now is a sex education syllabus which comes to terms with social reality.

EROTICISM AND SEXUALITY

A problem many adults face, even if they recognise that children are sexual throughout their entire life-span, is seen in the confusion and doubts raised by the term 'erotic'. It may be recognised that sexuality is not the sole monopoly of adolescents and adults, but eroticism applied to children raises many fears. The basic meaning of these words is based upon the Greek word *eros* for sexual love or desire. When we talk about behaviour being 'erotic' we usually associate it with sexual arousal, sexual desire and sexual satisfaction. Erotic songs, poems or pictures are said to evoke sexual drives and may lead to their fulfilment. For this reason many adults would reject the use of the word 'erotic' when applied to childhood.

The true picture of a child's sexual development reveals no clear-cut distinction between childhood and the later stages of life. It would be false to assert that some children's experiences are not erotic, since the evidence we have presented indicates arousal from a very early age, the existence of some kind of excitement and the desire for some kind of sexual fulfilment. Arousal may be in the form of sexual curiosity which is partly intellectual but it is also in the realm of feeling and emotion. To suggest that children are devoid of emotion in relation to their growing sexuality is to deny an important aspect of their development. Yet it is precisely this which frightens many adults and leads to repression of children's sexual growth.

We have already discussed in some detail the natural tendency of children to touch and explore their own bodies during babyhood and infancy. They derive not only comfort from this activity but also much pleasure. This may at first be experienced as sensual pleasure especially when the sex organ is touched and fondled, but because much of this is experienced with adults at bathtime, or when having nappies changed, it is also part of the emotional bonding with parents.

Yet when children themselves initiate touching and fondling of their own sex organ, adults generally find it difficult to accept. By body language, dissuasion and simple repression we tend to deny our children from a very early age the basic enjoyment of their sexual bodies.

Eroticism in the form of sexual arousal and the search for satisfaction does not arrive as some entirely new experience with the onset of adolescence. It has grown gradually through babyhood, infancy and childhood as the young interact with their own bodies, through lessons learned within the family and later in interaction with their peers. We do not know precisely when the erotic moves from the self to another love object, but it is probable that this takes place gradually in late childhood, as pubertal growth occurs over a number of years. Certainly the sensations experienced through the primary and secondary sex organs become more intense, and masturbation with a love object as part of sexual fantasy may begin. Older children develop crushes upon adored adults, often laughingly dismissed as 'puppy love'. These crushes are undoubtedly sexual in nature and precede the later sexual attractions recognised as having erotic meanings.

It is important then to recognise that sexuality throughout childhood does involve feelings of pleasure. Normal development involves these emotional experiences moving from the self to others in the family, to friends of the same age, and eventually becoming more overtly sexual during adolescence. If we are to meet the growing needs of children we must nourish this emotional development. Certainly limits have to be recognised where necessary, but gently and sensitively, rather than in a repressive manner.

MOVING BEYOND FREUDIAN THEORY

Theorists other than Sigmund Freud have written about childhood sexuality. But even such an encyclopedic investigator as Jean Piaget has dealt only briefly with sexual matters as perceived by children. He notes that when a child is told that a baby is inside the mother, the question then asked is 'Has she eaten it then?' Piaget also posits three stages by which children perceive the origin of babies. But he does not attempt an adequate theory to explain childhood sexuality. Kohlberg similarly concentrates, in his research on moral development, on how children perceive certain sexual situations containing a moral choice, but does not provide a comprehensive theory of childhood sexuality.[4]

It is the psychoanalysts following the works and writings of Sigmund Freud who have produced the only widely accepted theory of human sexuality. The most controversial of Freud's pronouncements was not the centrality of sex in human thought, emotion and behaviour, but the assertion of infantile sexuality, namely that humans are sexual and behave sexually from birth. Freud's theory, or rather theories, are often shrewd and brilliant in their description of human nature. Psychology and its related disciplines will be forever in Freud's debt for the new insights he provided into the realm of sexuality.

However, new evidence, much of it reported in this book, leads us to question a number of Freud's basic ideas. A broader theory, based upon research involving more normal samples of human beings, is needed and is in the process of emerging. One recognised limitation of Freud's theories is that they are based upon clinical cases, mostly involving neurosis. Moreover these cases are the product of an upper middle class mid-European society of the late nineteenth and early twentieth centuries. They are hardly typical of the population of modern and more varied democratic societies. What looked like universal truths about sexuality when they were first developed now appear to be outdated and invalid as generalisations about human nature.

Certain generalisations of Freud have stood the test of time and appear to be validated by much more modern research. 'Sexual life does not begin only at puberty but starts with clear manifestations soon after birth' is borne out by later medical and psychological evidence. And again, 'Sexual life comprises the function of obtaining pleasure from zones of the body – a function which is subsequently brought into the service of reproduction' is a universal truth that few would question today.

Freud's pronouncements had the capacity to shock particularly the prudish society of Vienna, of which he was a member. For example, 'We say that the human being has originally two sexual objects – himself [sic] and the woman who nurses him – and in doing so we are postulating a primary narcissism in everyone.'[5] Such statements were the beginnings of an elaborate theory, or a series of *ad hoc* theories, developed to order and explain clinical findings. Many of these theories were subject to considerable change, especially concerning childhood sexuality. It soon became evident that what patients report may not be actual happenings during childhood but may be the sexual fantasies of adults projected backwards into their earliest years. Not until the psychoanalytic approach was applied directly to children in play therapy by Anna Freud and Melanie Klein were theories of childhood sexuality more precisely formulated and systematised. Even so, these psychoanalytic theories are still imprecise and the basic ideas largely untested and unproven. To complicate matters further, post-Freudian analysts such as Eric Fromm and Karen Horney have advanced different theories and interpretations. Anthropologists such as Ruth Benedict and Margaret Mead have questioned the universality of Freudian theories in the light of sexual practices in varying societies and cultures.

In order to understand why the Freudian theory needs a critical reappraisal, we shall briefly describe it and see what in particular is being challenged by new evidence.[6]

Freud liberated the word 'sex' from its narrow copulatory meaning to a broader meaning which included any pleasurable sensation experienced by children, and strongly associated with eating (an oral stage), evacuating (an anal stage) and the genitals (a phallic stage). This later stage was seen to be repressed by children because of their anxiety, in the form of castration fears, that adults would punish them. Hence, according to Freud, guilt and neurosis have a sexual origin. This leads to what Freud termed 'the latency period' from about 4 years of age until about 10 or 11 years (the onset of puberty) when sexual interest and activity are suppressed so that psychosexual development slows down or becomes latent. Castration fears, Freud suggests, arise from the Oedipal situation in the family, where a boy perceives himself as the sexual rival of his father for the affections of the mother. For girls there is a so-called Electra complex, where the girl competes with her mother for the affection of her father. Freud posits the family as the scene of intense sexual conflict, accounting for sexual repression in the early and middle years of childhood.

There are four areas which are now being questioned even by psychoanalysts, although orthodox Freudians still defend them as valid. The first is the latency period. There is simply no evidence to show that children's sexual interests and activities diminish or abate during childhood. Indeed the evidence, including our own presented in this book, indicates a quite contrary development. Sexual interests and activities increase perceptibly in the years from 4 to 11. Certainly some of it becomes secretive, but this can be explained by general social inhibitions and children learning to observe limits, rather than by a dramatic sexual conflict within the family. And there is simply no evidence for widespread castration fears, which are said to inhibit sexual exploration.

Unfortunately, the practical effects of Freud's latency period have had a negative impact on the provision of sex education. It is frequently cited as the reason why sex education should not be given in the primary school years because the students' interests and activities are 'latent'. This flies in the face of the evidence and the urgent need of children for sex education programs, to prepare them for possible early maturing.

The second area to be questioned is Freud's later assertion that child sexual abuse in the form of incest is merely fantasy, arising from Oedipal rivalry, and is not in fact real. Early in his career Freud gave a paper based upon experiences with his first patients, positing actual incest in childhood as the origin of hysterical disorders. But he retracted this point of view and began to explain incest as fantasy, possibly to allay the criticisms of his colleagues.[7]

By relegating incest and similar child sexual abuse to fantasy Freud did a disservice to many generations of adults who as children had real experiences of this kind. The figures we have produced in Chapters 11 and 12 on the incidence of child molestation are disturbing. But by relegating such experiences to fantasy, Freud inadvertently puts the blame on the victim. It is the child who is the seducer, the sexual nymphomaniac, who desires the adult. This has had the effect of damning children, and girls especially, as liars and little Lolitas. Defending

251

lawyers in many incest cases which have come to trial have actually used these points. Even today many physicians, lawyers and other professionals tend to dismiss child sexual abuse and incest in particular as the product of childhood fantasy.

A third area of childhood sexuality theory advanced by Freud which needs questioning is his sketchy and unsatisfactory explanation of female sexuality. The description of the Electra complex seems to have been added as an afterthought by Carl Jung. The view that a girl's castration fears are based upon her perception that she has already been castrated for her sexual sins borders on the absurd. Freud's undoubted emphasis is upon male sexuality, and in many ways he reflects the sexism of his day in his writings.

The final area of Freud's theory to be questioned is his perception of homosexuality as an expression of sexual immaturity or 'arrested development'. For him the norm is for same-sex friendships to be superseded by other-sex friendship leading to full heterosexual relationships. In other words, homosexuals are regressive in their development and need to grow up. Part of this regression is to remain unduly attached to a parent well beyond childhood, or to retain narcissistic tendencies, characteristic of early stages of development. Freud's views are based on only one possible explanation of homosexuality, and has had the unfortunate consequence of a general assumption that homosexuality can be treated as a sickness. Again the evidence is to the contrary, and many homosexuals referred to psychologists, psychiatrists and psychoanalysts have been subjected to unnecessary and unhappy treatment.

What then is needed if much of Freud's theory now seems unacceptable and invalid in the light of evidence to the contrary? What is required is a theory which views sexuality through the whole span of life, and especially one which is consistent with the continuous and developing interests and activities of children. Physiological explanations of hormonal growth and the manifestation of earlier physical maturing are needed. The relationships between emotional, pleasurable and erotic experiences require exploration as do their links with intellectual perceptions of the self. A more adequate theory of developmental heterosexuality is required, with homosexuality seen in more normal perspective. And certainly the impact of the culture on how people perceive and control their sexuality by moral values is an important area to develop.

Theory is fundamentally an attempt to explain what we observe. We need broader and more valid explanations of the facts of human sexuality as more and more evidence comes to light. This would help us all to handle sex and sexuality more wisely, especially the sexual development of children and adolescents which so many find problematic. Theory can provide us with a framework within which parents and others can come to terms with and help children in their sexual growth to develop into well-rounded parents of the next generation.

NOTES AND REFERENCES

Preface

1   This is quoted in Wendy Lowenstein's book *Shocking, Shocking, Shocking: the Improper Play Rhymes of Australian Children* (Fish & Chips Press, Melbourne, 1974), but there are many more in Iona and Peter Opie's *The Lore and Language of Schoolchildren* (Paladin, London, 1977), Ian Turner's *Cinderella Dressed in Yella* (Heinemann, Melbourne, 1978) and June Factor's book *Children's Folklore*, to be published by Penguin Books, Australia, in 1988.

2   See the full report by Ronald and Juliette Goldman, *Children's Sexual Thinking* (Routledge & Kegan Paul, London, Boston and Melbourne, 1982).

3   Ronald and Juliette Goldman, *Family and Relations Survey* (Centre for the Study of Community, Education and Social Change, La Trobe University, Melbourne, 1986). This is a survey of children's sexual experiences.

4   See David Finkelhor, *Sexually Victimized Children* (Free Press, New York, 1979), and by the same author, *Child Sexual Abuse: New Theory and Research* (Free Press, New York, 1984).

Introduction

1   For both sexual and gender differences, Michael Carrera's book *Sex, the Facts, the Acts and Your Feelings* (Lansdowne, Sydney, London, New York, 1981) is excellent.

2   See Tom Bower's *Development in Infancy* (Freeman, San Francisco, 1982) and his *Perceptual World of the Child* (Harvard University Press, Cambridge, 1977).

3   J. M. Tanner's book *Foetus into Man* (Harvard University Press, Cambridge, 1978) gives some overall figures. The only reliable figures are from developed industrialised countries where health and other statistics have

been kept for several generations. Developing countries, because they lack the facilities, do not keep such figures. It is often assumed that children in tropical climates mature earlier than those in more temperate climates. But this may not be due to climate so much as the fact many countries in tropical zones have no or only limited industrialisation and are still operating agricultural peasant-type economies. Dr Tanner produces anecdotal evidence to suggest pre-Industrial Revolution children in Britain matured earlier than a century or more later. He argues that children in industrialised countries may only now be returning to the pre-industrial norm.

4　See Michael Carrera, *Sex, the Facts, the Acts and Your Feelings* and also *The Family Book About Sexuality* by Mary Calderone & Eric Johnson (Harper & Row, New York, 1981).

5　Tanner, *Foetus into Man*.

6　Schofield's book *The Sexual Behaviour of Young People* (Penguin, Harmondsworth, 1968) was followed by his later book *Promiscuity* (Gollancz, London, 1978). Another British report is Farrell's *My Mother Said* (Routledge & Kegan Paul, London, 1978). Some New Zealand figures are given in R. A. C. Stewart's *Adolescence in New Zealand* (Heinemann, Auckland, 1976).

7　The Alan Guttmacher Institute in New York has published *Teenage Pregnancy: the Problem That Hasn't Gone Away.* A similar report in Britain is *Pregnant at School* (National Council for One Parent Families, London, 1979). Also see Stewart, *Adolescence in New Zealand.*

8　See our survey of the Swedish syllabus, 'A Critical Evaluation of the Swedish (1977) Sex Education Syllabus', in the *Australian Journal of Sex, Marriage and Family*, August and November 1985.

9　Evidence for this can be seen in J. M. Masson's book *The Assault on Truth: Freud's Suppression of the Seduction Theory* (Farrar, Straus & Giroux, New York, 1984) and Janet Malcolm's *In the Freud Archives* (Flamingo Books, London, 1986).

10　L. L. Constantine & F. M. Martinson (eds), *Children and Sex: New Findings New Perspectives* (Little, Brown & Company, Boston, 1981).

11　See C. S. Ford & F. A. Beach's classic survey, *Patterns of Sexual Behaviour* (Harper & Row, New York, 1951).

1 How Sex Differences are Perceived

1 See the article by O. Pocs & A. Godow 'Can students view parents as sexual beings?', in *Family Co-ordinator* 26, 1977.

2 Stephanie Waxman's book was published by Widescope, Melbourne in 1976.

2 How are Babies Made?

1 See 'Children's awareness of the origin of babies', by J. H. Conn, in the *Journal of Child Psychiatry* 1, 1947, pp. 140-76.

2 A very readable account of this is given in *The Flight of the Stork* by Anne Bernstein (Delacorte, New York, 1978).

3 See Mary Calderone & Eric Johnson's *The Family Book About Sexuality* (Harper & Row, New York, 1981) p. 54.

4 See for example Per Holm Knudsen's picture book, *How a Baby is Made* (Piccolo, London and Sydney, 1980).

3 What Happens in Pregnancy and Childbirth?

1 Many of these books are inexpensive paperbacks and should be part of a family and school library. We could recommend Per Holm Knudsen's book *How a Baby is Made* and Peter Mayle's *Where Did I Come From?* (Sun, London and Melbourne, 1979) for young children. They explain conception, the various stages of pregnancy and childbirth. For older primary school children Christina Palmgren & Hilary Spiers *How You Are Made* (J. M. Dent, London, 1972) and Lennart Nilsson's *A Child Is Born* (Faber & Faber, London, 1980) are useful pictorial books with quite clear texts to be read by parents or teachers, or by older children themselves.

When buying these and other books, and there are many on the market, always check that the pictures are explicit and clear. Too many books show plenty of attractive pictures of babies and animals but are far too coy about the important facts of intercourse, conception and childbirth.

4 Sexual Intercourse and Sex Determination

1 W. H. Masters & V. E. Johnson, *The Pleasure Bond: A new look at sexuality and commitment* (Little, Brown, Boston, 1975). Alex Comfort's book

The Joy of Sex (Quartet Books, London, 1972) has been a very popular publication.

2   *The Facts of Love* (Mitchell Beazley, London, 1980) is written by Alex & Jane Comfort, and *Will I Like It?* (Hutchinson, Melbourne and W. H. Allen, London, 1978) is by Peter Mayle. These are both good straight-talking books, with humour and honesty, which do not minimise the problems and responsibilities involved in the sex act.

5   How Not to Have Babies

1   A British survey done by Michael Schofield was published as *The Sexual Behaviour of Young People* by Penguin Books in 1968. John Collins published an Australian survey 'Adolescent dating intimacy' in *Journal of Youth and Adolescence* 3 (4) in 1974. A Swedish survey by K. Sundstrom called 'Young people's sexual habits in today's Swedish society' is in *Current Sweden*, July 1976. An American survey called 'The sexual behaviour of adolescents in middle America' was published in the *Journal of Marriage and the Family* 34 in November 1972 by A. M. Venner, C. S. Stewart & D. L. Hager.

Michael Schofield's survey found that many boys thought they had had sexual intercourse and had practised withdrawal when in fact they had engaged in genital apposition, namely the rubbing of the penis against the external part of the girl's sex organ (the vulva) leading often to the boy's ejaculation. What most teenagers do not appear to know is that such an ejaculation may lead to a pregnancy even if penetration does not occur, since sperm may still find their way into the vagina and impregnate the girl's ovum.

2   See Michael Carrera's *Sex, the Facts, the Acts and Your Feelings*, page 60, for a discussion of IUDs, and pages 43-86 for full descriptions of all birth control methods.

3   See our survey of the Swedish syllabus, 'A Critical Evaluation of the Swedish (1977) Sex Education Syllabus', in the *Australian Journal of Sex, Marriage and Family*, August and November 1985.

6   Wearing Clothes and Being Naked

1   David Finkelhor wrote an unpublished paper called 'The Sexual Climate of Families' in 1980.

2 See note 3 to the Introduction.

3 These are known as instrumentalist and expressive theories, and are described by M. E. Roach & J. B. Eicher in their Book *Dress, Adornment and the Social Order* (John Wiley, New York, 1965).

4 See Lawrence Kohlberg's *Stages in the Development of Moral Thought and Action* (Holt, Rinehart & Winston, New York, 1969). Kohlberg writes about six stages and three levels. For details of this see our book *Children's Sexual Thinking*, Chapter 15.

5 See Sears, Maccoby & Levin's book *Patterns of Child Rearing* (Harper & Row, New York, 1957) and Newson & Newson's classic called *Four Years Old in an Urban Community* (Allen & Unwin, London, 1968).

6 In *Stages in the Development of Moral Thought and Action*.

7 What the Young Want to Know about Sex

1 See *World Health Statistics Annual* for statistics on 'Infectious diseases' published by the World Health Organisation.

2 Some of these situations are voiced by the children we interviewed, and others in Mary Calderone & James Ramey's book, *Talking With Your Child About Sex* (Random House, New York, 1982), an excellent book we recommend.

INTRODUCTION TO PART TWO

1 See our *Family and Relations Survey*.

8 Parents and Marriage

1 See B. Linner's two publications, *Sex and Society in Sweden* (Random House, New York, 1971) and her article 'No illegitimate children in Sweden', published in *Current Sweden* by the Swedish Institute in 1977.

2 See Patricia Edgar's *Children and Screen Violence* (University of Queensland Press, Brisbane, 1977).

9 Sexual Embarrassments in the Family

1 See the two Kinsey reports *Sexual Behaviour in the Human Male* (1948) and *Sexual Behaviour in the Human Female* (1953), both published by

Sanders, Philadelphia. Michael Carrera has a very sensible discussion of the topic in *Sex, the Facts, the Acts and Your Feelings.*

2   See Morton Hunt's *Sexual Behaviour in the 1970s* (Chicago, Playboy Press, 1974) and Sheryl Hite *The Hite Report* (New York, Dell, 1976).

3   Reported by Thore Langfeldt in *Children and Sex*, edited by Larry Constantine & Floyd Martinson (Little, Brown, Boston, 1981).

11   Children with Adults: Child Sexual Abuse

1   David Finkelhor pioneered this type of study, as reported in *Sexually Victimized Children.* This was replicated by a study of women students in Alabama by Dr Fromuth in her PhD thesis, and in Canada by three academics, Sorrenti-Little, Bagley & Robertson, as reported in the journal *Canadian Children* 9, 1984. Dr A. W. Baker & S. P. Duncan published an article reporting the prevalence of child sexual abuse in Britain in the *Journal of Child Abuse and Neglect* in 1986.

2   Some of these descriptions can be read in *Sexually Abused Children and Their Families*, edited by P. Mrazek and H. Kempe (Pergamon Press, Oxford, 1981).

3   A useful survey of studies in various countries, including those we cite, is made by David Finkelhor in his 1984 book *Child Sexual Abuse: New Theory and Research.*

4   We would recommend Freda Briggs' most useful book, called *Child Sexual Abuse: Confronting the Problem*, a paperback published by Pitman in 1986. Part 2 on 'Protective Education' is particularly clear and outlines what is needed in practical terms.

12   Children with Relatives: Incest

1   See J. Renvoize's book *Incest, a Family Pattern* (Routledge & Kegan Paul, London, 1982).

2   A very readable account of this theory and its consequences can be seen in Jeffrey Masson's book *The Assault on Truth: Freud's Suppression of the Seduction Theory.*

3   There have been exceptional cases where a child, or group of children, have falsely accused an adult of sexual abuse. Such cases are given considerable publicity in the press and create a completely wrong impression. These reports do not provide a valid argument that all

children's reports are the product of malicious intent or childish fantasy.

4   Dr Rosenfeld discusses 'Sleeping patterns in upper middle class families when the child awakens ill or frightened' in an article of this title in *Archives of General Psychiatry*, August 1982.

5   Such programs as Hank Giarretto's in California are outlined in some detail in the book *Sexually Abused Children and Their Families* edited by Patricia Mrazek & Henry Kempe.

13   First Sexual Experiences

1   Some very sensible advice on this topic is given by Jane Cousins in her award-winning book *Make It Happy*, published by Penguin Books in 1978. This book is a very useful one to buy for teenagers to read about many sexual matters.

2   Michael Schofield in his book *Promiscuity* (Gollancz, London, 1976) provides very convincing evidence about the young people he sampled being concerned with faithfulness in their sexual relationships.

3   A good discussion of the Swedish experience is given in Wendy McCarthy's and Sol Gordon's book *Raising Your Child Responsibly in a Sexually Permissive Society* (Collins, Sydney, 1984) in Chapter 5. This book is a very sensible guide for anxious parents.

4   See our 'Critical Evaluation of the Swedish (1977) Sex Education Syllabus' in the *Australian Journal of Sex, Marriage and Family* 6, 3 and 4 (1985).

5   Michael Carrera is one of the few writers on homosexuality to summarise the various theories, in *Sex, the Acts, the Facts and Your Feelings*. He lists several but points out that none of these is proven by research data, and that few are capable of being proved or disproved. There is the genetic theory, that homosexual orientation is decided by the genes. Then there is the hormone theory, that homosexuality is due to an imbalance of the sex hormones. There are three major psychoanalytic theories; that homosexuality is due to arrested development, same-sex parent attachment, or narcissistic tendencies. Finally there is the 'peer influence' theory, namely that peer pressure strongly influences sexual preferences.

We may add that these theories seek to explain practising homosexuals whose sole preference is the same sex. They do not, in our view, adequately explain the large number of bi-sexuals in our society.

6   We suggest that parents who are concerned about this situation refer to Michael Carrera's book *Sex, the Facts, the Acts and Your Feelings* and Jane Cousins' book *Make It Happy*. Both these are suitable to give to teenagers

to read. Many books provide contacts for gay support groups and further readings, as in *Young, Gay and Proud*, published by the Melbourne Gay Teachers and Students Group.

14 Helping Adults to Help Children

1 See Freud's 'The sexual researches of children' (1905), 'The sexual enlightenment of children' (1907) and 'On the sexual theories of children' (1908), published in *The Standard Edition of the Works of Sigmund Freud*, vols VI and IX (Hogarth Press, London).

2 Stevi Jackson's *Childhood and Sexuality* (Basil Blackwell, Oxford, 1982) provides a valuable discussion for parents and others.

3 These and related figures are reviewed in Chapter 2 of our book *Children's Sexual Thinking*.

4 See Michael Schofield's book *Promiscuity*.

5 R. Lewis in his article 'Parents and peers' in the *Journal of Sex Research* 9 (1973) reports on a valuable study of parents and their children.

6 See the work of Lawrence Kohlberg in *Stages in the Development of Moral Thought and Action*.

7 The Peter Mayle series (see note 1, Chapter 3 and note 2, Chapter 4) is useful but the best we can recommend is Mary Calderone and James Ramey's book *Talking With Your Child About Sex*. Its subtitle is 'Questions and Answers for Children from Birth to Puberty'.

8 See our suggestions for a basic library for home and school (note 1, Chapter 3).

15 Some Difficult and Unresolved Issues

1 *Instruction Concerning Interpersonal Relations* (National Swedish Board of Education, Stockholm, 1977; English translation 1982).

2 We have already mentioned *Young, Gay and Proud* published by the Melbourne Gay Teachers and Students Group. Gay contacts are also given as mentioned earlier in McCarthy & Gordon's *Raising Your Child Responsibly in a Sexually Permissive Society*.

3 We would recommend Dennis Altman's *Homosexual: Oppression and Liberation* (Penguin, Melbourne, 1971); B. Fairchild & N. Hayward's *Now That You Know: What Every Parent Should Know About Homosexuality* (Harcourt, Brace, Jovanovich, New York, 1979); J. J. MacNeill's *The Church*

and the Homosexual (Pocket Books, New York, 1976).

4 See Piaget's *The Child's Conception of the World* (1929) and Kohlberg's *Stages in the Development of Moral Thought and Action*.

5 All the quotations from Freud are taken from the *Standard Edition* of his works.

6 An admirable overview can be read in J. A. C. Brown's *Freud and the Post-Freudians* (Penguin, Harmondsworth, 1961).

7 This particular action of Freud is explored in Jeffrey Masson's book *The Assault on Truth: Freud's Suppression of the Seduction Theory*. It is now in paperback.

INDEX

abnormal sexual play of children, 162-3

Aboriginal girls, 201

abortion, xxviii, 3, 71, 74-8, 222, 237, 238, 239

abstention from sex, 81, 206

abusers, 168-70, 179, 185, 219

Adam and Eve, 90, 95

adolescence, xxvi, 5, 11, 19, 94, 167, 188, 193, 201, 215, 220, 221, 228, 240-4, 257

adoption, 71, 73, 238

afterbirth, 52, 55

age of consent, 165

ageing and sex, 121, 134

'agriculturalists', 25-6, 35

AIDS (Acquired Immune Deficiency Syndrome), xxviii, 88, 112, 213, 240-4, 246

alcoholism, 124, 173, 180, 185

ALTMAN, Dennis, 261

amniotic sac, 46

anal stage, 250

androgyny education, 18

animalculism, 28

animals in sex education, 34, 62

anthropology, xxx, 89, 190

babies
    newborn, xiv, xx, xxii, 5
    origin of, 21-37, 108-9, 215, 223, 232, 256
    sexual activity of, xxi

Baby factories, 24

BAKER, Tony, 175

basal body temperature (bbt) method of contraception, 83

bathroom etiquette 137, 140-1

BAKER, A. W., 259

BEACH, F. A., 255

belly button, 26, 43, 49, 58, 108

BENEDICT, Ruth, 250

BERNSTEIN, Anne, 256

Bible, sex in the, 128

birth control see contraception

birth exit, 47-51, 55-6, 57

bisexuals, 207, 260

books to use for sex education, 18, 34, 56, 61-2, 231, 246, 256-7

BOWER, Tom, 254

breasts
    growth of, xxvi, 9, 19, 107, 201, 202
    size of, 98

BRIGGS, Freda, 179, 259

BROWN, J. A. C., 262

Caesarean section, xi, 39, 48, 51, 56

Caesarean theory of conception, xi, 52

CALDERONE, Mary, 255, 258, 261

CARRERA, Michael, 208, 244, 254, 255, 257, 259, 260

castration, 83, 250-2

Catholics, Roman, 145, 237, 243

chastity, 239

child pornography, xiii, xv, xxx, 229

child sexual abuse, xv, xxix, xxx, 101, 142, 162, 164-79, 218, 220, 241, 251, 259
    international comparisons, 175-6, 220
    preventive programs, 162, 177, 192

childbirth, xxiv, 3, 46-57, 58, 71

children's sexual experiences
    with adults, 164-79
    with children, 148-63
    with relatives, 180-94

children's hostility for the other sex, 16-18, 19

children's sexual preferences, 13-16

chromosomes, xix, 29, 68, 223

clergy, 48, 65

clitoris, 198

clothes, reasons for wearing, 89-101 *see also* modesty training

coitus interruptus, 30, 82

COLLINS, John, 257

COMFORT, Alex, 256, 257

conception, xvii, xxviii, 28, 32, 36, 52, 71, 108-9, 203

condoms, 84-7, 110, 241, 242, 243

conformity to social convention, 91-4

CONN, J. H., 256

consensus morality, 91, 94-5

CONSTANTINE, L. L., 255

contraception, xxviii, 29, 71, 72, 78, 86, 109-10, 112, 188, 206, 237, 239, 240

contraceptive devices, 84-6, 240, 243

courtship behaviour, 111, 112

cousins, 152-3, 169, 174, 180

COUSINS, Jane, 260

curiosity, xxiv, 56, 148-63, 200, 218, 227, 229, 231

dating, 195, 204-6, 208

death, 173, 242

deception about sex, 104, 213, 216-19, 231

diaphragm, 84-6

digestive fallacy, 25, 27, 35, 51, 57, 66

dirty language, xx, 69, 128, 227, 230

dirty jokes, 109, 140-1

divorce, 3, 12, 81, 123, 173, 222, 237

DNA, 68

doctors, xviii, 5, 39, 49, 52, 64, 65, 77, 79

DUNCAN, S. P., 259

Dutch cap *see* diaphragm

earlier maturing of children, xxvi, xxviii, 106, 196, 213, 222, 240

early developers, xxv, 104, 204, 236

Edinburgh University, xxii

EDGAR, Patricia, 258

eggs, 25-6, 27, 34, 58, 77, 108

EICHER, J. B., 258

ejaculation, 174, 197, 203, 204, 257

Electra complex, 250-2

elementary school *see* primary

embryo, 46, 63, 223
encyclopedias, 33, 109, 115, 128, 231
equality of the sexes, 18
erections, xxi, 9, 99
erotic, 157, 199, 247, 252
ethnic, diversity and sex education, 236, 238-9
exhibitionism, 154, 167, 169, 187
ex-nuptial births, xxviii, 132, 239

FACTOR, June, 254
FAIRCHILD, B., 261
fallopian tube, 45, 83
FARRELL, Christine, 255
fertilisation, xix, 64, 69
fetus, xxi, 42, 45, 46, 63, 223
father
    roles 9, 91, 170
    and child abuse, 170, 172, 173, 183, 184, 187
    see also parents
films, 3, 115
FINKELHOR, David, ix, 172, 182, 254, 257, 259
first sexual intercourse, xxvii, 30, 196, 206-7, 240, 241
folklore, children's, xii
force, in sexual encounters, 157, 170-1, 178, 238
FORD, C. S., 255
fostering, 71, 73
FREUD, Anna, 250
FREUD, Sigmund, xvi, xxi, xxix, 150, 189, 214, 218, 248-50, 261, 262
Freudian theory, 63, 189, 214, 237, 248-50
FROMM, Eric, 250
FROMUTH, M. E., 259

gay, 208, 214, 244-6

gender, xviii, xix, xx, xxiii, 10-11, 238
genes, 68, 223
genital apposition, xxvii, 155, 167, 257
genitals, 93, 148, 150, 154, 166, 169, 174, 180, 183, 222
'geographers', 22-5, 35
gestation, 41, 42, 71, 110
GIARRETTO, Hank, 193, 260
God, 23, 24, 36, 43, 60, 64, 79, 80
GODOW, A., 256
GOLDMAN, Ronald & Juliette, 254
gonorrhoea, xxviii
GORDON, S., 260, 261
grandfathers, 183, 187
Guttmacher Institute, xxviii, 255

HAYWARD, N., 261
hermaphroditism, xviii, xix
herpes, xxviii, 112, 213
Hite Report, 144, 199
homophilia, 15, 19, 205, 208
homosexuality, 15, 127, 195, 205, 207-12, 213, 238, 241, 244-6, 252-3, 260
homosexuals, sex education of, 244-6
honesty with children, 35, 231-3, 236
hormones, xviii, 68, 84, 252, 260
HORNEY, Karen, 250
hospitals, as source of babies, 24, 32, 36, 73, 79
HUNT, Morton, 259
hysterectomy, 83
hysterotomy, 51

illegitimacy, 132, 258
incest, xii, xxi, xxix, 12, 153, 180-94, 251

incestuous relationships, 181, 184, 186, 188, 190

Industrial Revolution, xxvii, 173, 255

intra-familial sexual experiences, 170, 181-8

IUDs (intra-uterine devices), 84-6

JACKSON, Stevi, 219, 261

Jesus, 23, 47, 64

Jews, 145, 237

JOHNSON, Eric, 255, 258

JOHNSON, V. E., 256

JUNG, Carl, 252

KEMPE, H., 259, 260

kindergarten, xxiv, 116, 152

KINSEY, Alfred C., 144, 199, 258

kissing, xxi, 27, 36, 124, 135, 138-9, 148, 154, 174, 205

KLEIN, Melanie, 250

KNUDSEN, Per, 256

KOHLBERG, Lawrence, 92, 248, 258, 261, 262

labour, 52, 54 see also childbirth

Labor Day, 47, 54

LANGFELDT, Thore, 259

latency period, 150, 250-1

lesbian, 208, 209, 246

LEVIN, 258

LEWIS, R., 261

LINNER, B., 258

love-making, 58, 136, 222

LOWENSTEIN, Wendy, 254

low-income families, 172, 185

MACCOBY, 258

MACNEILL, J. J., 261

male dominance, 14, 170

MALCOLM, Janet, 255

'manufacturers', 24-5, 35, 66, 71, 80

Maori girls, 201

marriage, xi, xviii, xxvii, 3, 60, 81, 121, 123-36, 185, 186, 222

MARTINSON, Floyd, 146, 255

MASSON, Jeffrey, 255, 259

MASTERS, W. H., 256

masturbation, xii, xxiii, 111, 118, 126, 127, 128, 143-5, 148, 151, 157, 161, 162, 164, 166, 183, 197-9, 200, 203, 226, 227, 237, 246

MAYLE, Peter, 57, 256, 257, 261

McCARTHY, W., 260, 261

MEAD, Margaret, xxxi, 250

meiosis, 45

menarche, 118, 198, 201-2, 204, 219

menstruation, xxv, xxvi, 9, 10, 30, 82, 105-7, 116, 187, 196, 201-2, 226, 237, 241

mentally handicapped, rights of, 239

'miniaturists', 27-8, 33, 64, 68, 217

modesty training, xii, xxv, 92, 100, 140, 159, 187, 227

morality, 90, 160, 213, 225-7, 236-40

mother
    roles, 91, 170
    and child abuse, 172, 173, 183-4, 185-7
    see also parents

MRAZEK, P., 259, 260

Muslims, 237-9

myths about conception, 29-30

nakedness, xxv, 4, 89-101, 137, 139-40, 186

natural (rhythm) methods of contraception, 82, 239

navel, 27, 43, 49
neonates *see* babies, newborn
New Zealand, xxvii, xxviii, 201, 207, 255
NILSSON, Lennart, 256
nocturnal emissions *see* wet dreams
normal sexual development, xiii, 161-2, 196-7
Norway, 146
nurses, xviii, 5, 48, 65, 77, 79

Oedipal complex, xiii, 189, 250, 251
OPIE, Iona & Peter, 254
oral sex, 82, 162, 167
oral stage, xxi, xxiv, 250
orphanages, 71, 73
ovaries, 84
ovism, 28
ovulation, 30, 84
ovum, 27, 28, 29, 34, 36, 232

Pacific Islanders, xxxi
PALMGREN, Hilary, 256
parents, 6, 64
    and child sexual abuse, 169, 180, 185, 187, 191-4, 231
    and sex education, 56-7, 104, 176-9, 180, 202, 203-4, 215-34
    as role models and authority figures, 91, 158-63, 185, 186, 195, 200-1
    attitudes to children's sexuality, xxx, 213, 216-19
    of homosexuals, 209-10
    roles in procreation, gestation, delivery, xii, 24-9, 30-7, 39, 41-6, 58
    sexuality of, 10-12, 125-6, 133-6
parenting, 111, 112-13

pederasty, xxix
pedophiles, xv, xxix, 229
penis, xx, xxii, xxv, 7, 18, 27, 105, 117, 160, 230
periods, 30, 99, 106 *see also* menarche, menstruation
pessaries, 84
phallic stage, 250
physically handicapped, rights of, 239
PIAGET, Jean, 248, 262
pill, the, 71, 76, 84-6, 242
placenta, 45, 46
play groups, xxiv
POCS, O., 256
police, 159, 173, 175
pregnancy, xi, xxiv, xxviii, 3, 21, 28, 35, 38-46, 56, 58, 110, 149, 215, 223, 232
    unwanted, 29, 238
primary school, xxiv, xxxi, 70, 116-17, 177, 198, 222, 242, 251
privacy, need for, 101, 238
procreation, 30-2, 61
promiscuity, 206, 207
Protective Child Sexual Abuse Programs, 101
psychoanalysts, xxiv, 189, 249-52
pubertal growth and changes, xxiv, xxvi, 8-10, 19, 104, 117, 167, 196, 201, 204, 224, 228, 232, 236, 242, 248, 250, 251
punishment, avoidance of, 91-3, 96-7, 197

RAMEY, J., 261
rape, 166, 190
'realists', 28-9, 33
religion, 23, 90, 236-40, 243
RENVOIZE, J., 259

reproduction, xvii, xviii, xxx, 3, 155, 188, 201, 215, 221, 222, 224, 226, 229, 249
ROACH, M. E., 258
ROSENFELD, Dr, 260
ROUSSEAU, Jean-Jacques, xxx
rural children, 172, 185

safety houses, 178
San Francisco, 175
SCHOFIELD, Michael, 224, 233, 255, 257, 260, 261
SEARS, 258
secondary schools, xxxi, 70, 103, 116, 223
seduction, 156, 184
seduction theory, 189-91, 251-2, 255
seed, 25-6, 34, 40, 66, 108, 232
self-pleasuring, 111, 197
semen, 203
sex
    definition of, xvii
    determination, 4, 62-70, 223
    differences, xviii, xxii, 5-20, 58, 105-6, 215, 223, 237
    education, xxvi, xxix, xxviii, xxxi, 4, 8, 33, 59, 70, 86, 102, 113, 115-17, 135, 177, 201, 207, 214, 220, 222, 224, 225, 228, 233-4, 238, 242
    games, xii, xxv, 127, 142, 148, 154-7, 182, 186, 191
    organs, xx, xxii, xxiii, xxv, 7, 18, 33, 34, 89, 95, 96-100, 104, 105, 128, 141, 149, 153, 161, 174, 177, 186, 217, 223, 230, 243
sexual embarrassments, 137-47
sexual enjoyment, 60-1
sexual experiences of children, 120-210, 215

sexual exploration, xxiii, 148-63, 182, 199
sexual fantasies, 144, 148, 155, 161, 189, 190, 199, 248, 250
sexual fondling, 154, 156, 161, 166, 167, 174, 182, 183, 187, 205, 247
sexual identity, xix, xx, xxiii, 5, 226
sexual innocence, xvii, xxx, 35, 177, 217, 221, 242
sexual intercourse, xi, xvii, xxx, 27, 29, 32, 33-35, 51, 58-62, 87, 109, 125, 126, 135, 155, 156, 166, 182, 196, 206-7, 215, 239, 243
sexual joining, 26, 36, 126, 135, 223, 242
sexual limits for children, 230-1, 248
sexual models, 135, 136, 188
sexual myths about children, 220-7
sexual myths of children, xii, 22, 35, 57, 104, 145, 213
sexual rivalry, xxx
sexual thinking, xiv, 1-118, 215
sexual vocabulary, xviii, xxii, 9
sexually transmitted diseases, xxviii, 111, 117, 213, 240-4
siblings, xxiii, 7, 143, 152, 158, 180, 182, 183, 191
sin, xxx, 144, 160, 237
slow developer, 104, 236
sperm, 28, 29, 32, 36, 67, 108, 232, 242
spermicides, 84
SPIERS, Christina, 256
stepfathers, 173, 180
STEWART, R. A. C., 255
'stranger danger', xii, 168, 169, 172, 178, 219

suckling, xxi
SUNDSTROM, K., 257
Sweden, xiii, xxvii, xxix, 4, 7, 15,
    32, 75, 79, 86, 87, 132, 220,
    223, 237
Swedish
    Family Planning Association,
    206
    National Board of Education,
    228, 261
    syllabus, xxix, 207, 229, 255,
    257
syphilis, xxviii, 111

taboos, 7, 34, 90, 96, 99, 125,
    128, 141, 151, 153, 186, 187,
    190
teachers, 115, 159, 198, 201, 224
TANNER, James M., 254
teenage pregnancy, xxviii, xxix,
    87, 176, 207, 220, 225, 240,
    243, 255
television, 3, 33, 43, 52, 71, 115,
    156, 222
thumb-sucking, xxiii, 197, 198
toilet training, xxii, xxiii, 92

transvestites, xix
TURNER, Ian, 254

umbilical cord, 46, 49, 83
uncles, 181, 184, 187
United Nations, 65
unwanted babies, 72-4
urethra, 50
urination, xx, 6, 7, 34, 150, 164
uterus, 22, 56

vagina, xx, xii, xxv, 7, 18, 27, 50,
    55, 105
vasectomy, 83, 84
venereal diseases, xxix, 88, 176,
    220, 229
VENNER, A. M., 257
vulva, 50, 198, 257

WAXMAN, Stephanie, 18
weaning, xxiv
wet dreams, xxv-vi, 107, 111,
    118, 196, 202-4, 219, 241
womb, xxi, 22, 36, 46, 51, 56, 77
WORLD HEALTH ORGANISA-
    TION, xxv, xxviii, 258